D1246528

"As someone who has been 'working with kundalini' for more than forty years now, I can tell you that this book is a must-read for anyone who has experienced kundalini or spiritual awakening. It is clear, pragmatic, and incredibly in-depth. It is very clear that Mary has the lived experience of kundalini to be able to guide others, and I am grateful that her compassionate, no-nonsense wisdom is available for those seeking insight and depth in their own process."

— FRANK KRIEGER, PH.D., philosopher and alchemist

"This extraordinary book is a no-nonsense guide to the unfurling process of kundalini energy. With straightforward narrative Mary shares her personal experiences with kundalini and its effects on her life while weaving in vastly researched knowledge of the process. Compassionate and thoughtful, this book is an essential guide to kundalini awakening."

— KATHY TAJIK, CEO of Tajik Home

"A clear, grounded, and balanced guide that provides a bridge between the everyday and the transcendental, offering a structured framework and practical suggestions without reducing the beauty of kundalini to a clinical process. As someone going through kundalini awakening, it spoke to both the parts of me that are discombobulated by this experience and to the part of me that knows, helping me to reorient myself on my path with greater clarity and trust."

— CHARLOTTE SAUNDERS, spiritual practitioner

"*Working with Kundalini* is a collection of field notes from a reliable, experienced guide who has shared her forays into the various states of being that denote our spiritual realities. It's a lucid, unpretentious, unvarnished, and thorough account of the phenomenon of kundalini experiences. Mary Shutan is reliable, because it's clear that she's done her own rigorous fieldwork on the subject. She brings to the forefront the nuances of states of awakening without trafficking in textbook claims of what this means. If anything, this book is an experiential journey into the most intimate and epic frontiers of consciousness. To read it is to get a direct taste of that."

— NIRMALA NATARAJ, editor, writer, and author of *Earth and Space* and *The Planets*

WORKING WITH
KUNDALINI

An Experiential Guide to the
Process of Awakening

MARY MUELLER SHUTAN

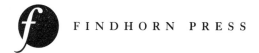
FINDHORN PRESS

Findhorn Press
One Park Street
Rochester, Vermont 05767
www.findhornpress.com

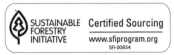

Text stock is SFI certified

Findhorn Press is a division of Inner Traditions International

Disclaimer

The information in this book is given in good faith and is neither intended to diagnose
any physical or mental condition nor to serve as a substitute for informed medical
advice or care. Please contact your health professional for medical advice and treatment.
Neither author nor publisher can be held liable by any person for any loss or damage
whatsoever which may arise from the use of this book or any of the information therein.

Cataloging-in-Publication Data for this title is available from the Library of Congress

ISBN 978-1-62055-881-2 (print)
ISBN 978-1-62055-882-9 (ebook)

Printed and bound in the United States by Lake Book Manufacturing Inc.
The text stock is SFI certified. The Sustainable Forestry Initiative® program promotes
sustainable forest management.

10 9 8 7 6 5 4 3 2 1

Edited by Jane Ellen Combelic
Cover design by Richard Crookes
Text design and layout by Damian Keenan
This book was typeset in Adobe Garamond Pro, Calluna Sans, Museo with
ITC Century Std Book Condensed and Trajan Pro used as display typefaces

To send correspondence to the author of this book, mail a first-class letter to the
author c/o Inner Traditions • Bear & Company, One Park Street, Rochester,
VT 05767, and we will forward the communication, or contact the author directly at
http://maryshutan.com

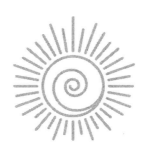

Contents

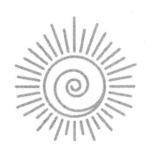

Introduction

Many people in our world today are going through some form of spiritual awakening. Some of these may be kundalini awakenings—the path of uniting our individual consciousness with cosmic intelligence. Such awakenings allow us to meet our full potential, to release past trauma, and to move beyond the conditionings of history and society. As the awakened flow of consciousness uncoils and rises through the midline, we evolve beyond the false self and the illusions of this world into an experience of oneness. This experience of oneness paradoxically leads to the realization of our individual divine potential.

Such awakenings are difficult for even the ready and stable soul, and vapid romanticism or horror stories are often found instead of a realistic view of the difficulties and joys of such an experience. While any pragmatic eye could look towards spiritual communities and see deep flaws, especially the usage of the spiritual path to further self-obsession and unhealthy patterns of relating, we have schismatically divided ourselves from the spiritual realms and any type of direct gnosis. Serious, nuanced consideration of what it means to directly experience spirit in our modern culture has become seriously endangered.

In a world so deeply split off from spirit, any experience beyond what is considered normal human existence becomes pathologized. Individuals who feel a deep call towards spirit or who experience spiritual awakenings find themselves confronted by society's deep fear of any type of direct revelation of the divine.

In our culture of scientific materialism, the idea that body, emotions, mind, and spirit are on a continuum, and that our material world is simply the densest and most noticeable aspect of that continuum, may never be appreciated. We have such complexity and depth as humans, yet we are only seen for a fraction of what we truly are.

We are spirit. We are consciousness. It is by connecting to something greater than ourselves that we realize what we are here to do and who we are meant to be. We are so disconnected today from ourselves, from other humans, from nature, from the divine. This type of disconnection is becoming normalized to the point where we are forgetting that we can be connected.

We are meant to be in a state of interbeing, a state of communion with those around us. And we realize on some level that we used to connect more deeply and authentically to the world around us. Connectivity is essential for our health and well-being, and we deeply feel the emptiness and lack of connection in our modern world.

Spiritual awakening involves looking directly at what is not working in our lives, how we are disconnected, how we may be unclear. On some level, we always know what lies unhealed within us, what is preventing us from being authentic and connected and vital in this world. It is only by looking directly at what disconnects us that we awaken.

The scientific materialist worldview seeks to quiet us, to numb what is uncomfortable or distressing. The idea that spiritual awakening is one of the most difficult things that we can experience, involving both pain and bliss, is something that the weary, modern soul is unwilling to contend with. Most of us are looking for a fast, simple solution to all of our pain. We consider "spiritual" to mean elevated, to mean some place where we no longer experience anything that may distress us. The end of suffering sounds nice to anyone, myself included. So does being in eternal bliss, or emptiness, or infinite love. So does the end of the inevitable ups-and-downs of our daily human struggle, or not having to contend with a rather messy and deteriorating human form that is deeply fearful of old age and death. From this vantage point, emotions and human experiences are to be anesthetized instead of celebrated, suppressed instead of allowed to flow.

We awaken by looking within, by becoming increasingly conscious and accepting of every aspect of ourselves. It is by deeply feeling our emotions and by accepting all aspects of ourselves as valid that we can awaken. We can access our light only if we truly know and accept our darkness. This path allows us to feel more, not less. It allows us to move beyond blind emotive reacting, beyond basic self-obsession. Thus we begin to see and sense more than ourselves: our family, our community, ancestry, society, the world, the cosmos. Moving beyond the self allows us to truly and deeply feel for others, because we see that what is in the world is also within ourselves.

Many of us are awakening in small and large ways in this world. Yet there is a distinct lack of nuanced information regarding spiritual awakenings. Whether it is called kundalini, chu'lel, n/um, Holy Spirit, cosmic energy, the interplay of Shiva and Shakti, spirit fire, orgasmic energy, creative energy, sambogakaya, cosmic healing force, the energy of liberation, or evolutionary energy, there have been accounts of people from all walks of life going through the kundalini awakening process for as long as we have accounts of the spiritual path in written form.

These accounts point to distinct experiences that are common to those who have awakened this energy in their systems, or in whom it may be emerging. They also describe the plethora of illusions present; it is part of the path to see those illusions, which can be quite tantalizing, and to go beyond them.

There are many gatekeepers in this world. In older spiritual traditions concepts like kundalini would be deliberately obscured or closely guarded, offered only to students who were ready for them. Nowadays, we have so much information at our fingertips—in moments we can access the profound spiritual writings on Kashmir Shaivism and Vedanta and then an account by a Christian mystic, all describing the kundalini awakening process. But there is so much information that we are lost in a great sea of noise, and it is an initiatory process in itself to find authentic or helpful information within that sea.

Over the years I have found immense help and support in discussions of kundalini emerging from many different cultures and understandings, especially Kashmir Shaivism, Hermeticism, different forms of Buddhism, Sufism, Vedanta, and Esoteric Christianity. Like many people who walk this path, I first found Gopi Krishna to be a gatekeeper to deeper knowledge of this process; Irina Tweedie's accounts were immensely helpful in understanding my own. It can be quite odd to see something that you have experienced written about by someone from a much different time and place. This is how it was for me when I came across some passages in *Interior Castle* by St. Teresa of Avila (published in 1577).

In the West we are experiencing a type of spiritual orphaning that has not become fully conscious or contended with by us. We tend to reach for other cultures and their mythologies and spiritual paths in an attempt to heal this. However, without long-term dedication to the path and full immersion in the daily reality and language of the culture, as well as under-standing the myths and the stories of that culture, much of the meaning becomes lost, romanticized, or obscured. We attempt to fit spiritual tradi-tions into a psychological framework because it fits into our modern, West-ernized sensibilities. In doing so we have lost contact with spirit, and how to discern between spiritual truth and mental creation.

The real difficulty in writing a book about kundalini is to do it simply, yet with the depth and reverence it deserves, and in a modern context that can be readily understood by the Western reader.

Students and clients over the years have told me that when looking for information they found three things: horror stories from people who were reportedly going through kundalini awakenings, information from a different culture or time that was too far out of context for them, and information from a psychological viewpoint. Upon further research they found good information from yogis regarding the technicalities of the process. They also came across the typical illusions from people promising that kundalini awakening means that they will never have to experience any issue in their lives again, or that such an awakening can be easily bought, sold, or experienced by anyone with little or no effort.

When this energy erupted within me I was twenty-three years old. For the next ten years I went through an intensive process, during which I could have used the guidance that I offer in these pages. Fifteen years after this initial eruption, my outlook on kundalini is quite different. I found through my studies that most of the information regarding kundalini is like a bad game of *Telephone*, the child's game where one person has information and passes it to the next person, and so on down the line until at the end the message has lost all meaning.

Kundalini awakening is not just a spiritual process. It is also not simply a psychological process, to be treated through psychotherapeutic means. Labeling the process as pathological because it does not adhere to societal norms is missing the point. It is also a physiological process, a rewiring that has a profound effect on the physical body, as well as the mind and spirit.

Kundalini awakening is our inherent birthright. It is not a pathological experience, but one that bestows great healing and expanded consciousness. It is a path that allows us to bring the totality of our authentic selves into the world. It is a path of great creativity, of awareness, which moves us beyond basic human selfishness to being of benefit in some small or large way to this world. It can also create a great deal of difficulty, pain, and emotional upheaval. Understanding what a kundalini awakening is and how it emerges takes us beyond pathologizing, romanticizing, or villainizing it. If we can see it as consciousness arising we can better help those who are experiencing it to make their way through the process.

This work is intended to be an in-depth, nuanced look at what happens in the modern kundalini process. It is for those who are experiencing a kundalini awakening process, or those who feel unsure if they are or not, as well as their family and friends. It is also for clinicians of all types who are willing to open their minds to see that there are many people going through profound, life-changing spiritual experiences that drastically affect every aspect of their being—mind, body, and spirit.

My viewpoint differs in some ways from what is commonly shared by others currently writing on this topic. This is because of my direct experience of this process, my own spiritual aptitude, and my work with clients going through spiritual awakenings over the last fifteen years, as well as extensive education in a variety of holistic, therapeutic, occult, and spiritual disciplines. These have taken me to some rather odd depths in an effort to understand my own experiences, and have led me to be of benefit to others in theirs.

This book explains what kundalini is, how it emerges, and the different phases of kundalini awakening. It offers guidance around diet and lifestyle, herbal supplements and herbal allies. How to find help and what healing work and methods may be of assistance make up the last section of the book. Also included is a list of books that were most useful in my personal understanding of the process.

To all those snake-bitten, I welcome you to a path of immense healing, wholeness, bliss, difficulty, pain, and wonder.

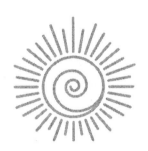

1

My Story

I remember being six years old and going to the Chicago Art Institute and seeing Georges Seurat's *A Sunday Afternoon on the Island of La Grande Jatte*. After my father explained that the artwork was called pointillism—a series of dots coming together to create the scene—I would sit on the couch and consider myself as a series of dots, and wonder what would happen if those dots began to come apart. I had dreams of being in water and dissolving into a series of dots that would become waves. Such dreams and revelations were not terrifying, but felt pleasurable and I always woke up in a heightened, flowing state that lasted for hours.

I was always someone who deeply felt, and who was quite sensitive and open. There was little context for this in the world I grew up in; much of my behavior and way of relating to the world was explained away through my artistic sensibilities. I was also deeply connected to nature; I was immensely happy in Minnesota where I would commune with the birch trees and the small lake behind my house. I didn't understand until years later why I became so unhappy when my family moved to a suburb that had little to no nature.

From an early age I was interested in folklore, fairy tales, mythology, as well as witchcraft, the supernatural, and the occult. But it didn't occur to me until I was in my mid-twenties that these were "spiritual" topics. For me "spiritual" was a far-off memory of attending church a few times.

My parents were intellectuals who fostered my love of reading. I feel a lot of gratitude towards them that they let me read whatever I wanted to or could manage to check out from the local library. But while they encouraged any type of education or literature, my parents did not bring religious or spiritual topics of discussion into the household, and are not mystical or terribly sensitive people.

I grew up knowing that there was something distinctly Other about me. In many ways I was a typical child—I had friends, did well on my schoolwork when I cared to put effort into it, and went through many of the typical initiations of childhood and adolescence. But in other ways I grew up fearing that something was deeply wrong with me, or that people would find out that there was something wrong with me.

I was always curious and open to those who were also Othered by the world in some capacity. In them I hoped to find the key to what was Other within myself. I was lucky to grow up in a household that had a lot of different types of books, and at an early age I read books like *Gone with the Wind*, *Night* by Elie Wiesel, and *The Autobiography of Malcolm X* (at the age of ten I was more enamored with the description of wearing zoot suits by Malcolm X than any of his more notable achievements).

As a teenager I was fascinated by the grotesque eloquence of Joyce Carol Oates and the magical realism of writers like Isabel Allende, Umberto Eco, and Gabriel Garcia Marquez. They spoke to a world that was completely internal for me at that age. While my parents and community were solidly middle class (or at times upper middle class) my environment lacked any sort of emotional depth. I learned quite quickly that my books, artwork, writing, and piano playing were appropriate outlets for my emotions, but expressing my sensitivity was seen as wrong. If I expressed my grief, anger, or joy through a painting, it was put up in the school and I was told how wonderful it was. If I won a writing award, I was praised. But if I allowed myself to vitally express my emotions through my physical form, I was sent to the counselor. This was incredibly confusing for me as a child, and although I understand it now as an adult, it still points to huge societal problems with emotional intelligence and our need to placate, medicate, or suppress any form of emotional expression in our culture.

I had some wonderful teachers who nurtured my love of books and the way that I perceived the world, and who were sympathetic to my difficulties. But I still had immense difficulties at school as I was in a continual state of overwhelm and exhaustion from being so open and sensitive.

My spiritual experiences began to intensify in my teenage years, and in my late teens I began to have intensive *shamanic dismemberment dreams* involving being devoured by snakes. Shamanic dismemberment dreams are dreams or visions of being devoured, dismembered, torn apart, or dissolved. They point psychologically to a process of death and rebirth, specifically a disintegration of identity followed by the formulation of a new one.

In spiritual terms such dreams are one of the first callings of someone who is intended to do work of a spiritual nature for their community. If you had asked me previous to the age of twenty-three what I wanted to do with my existence, I would have said that I wanted to be a writer. Specifically a novelist and poet, and this had been a continual interest for me ever since my mother would bring out her typewriter and type out my poems and stories for me at age six. While becoming a writer is still a core aspect of who I am, kundalini awakening has led me down a much different path than I once anticipated for myself.

Kundalini Emerges

I used to say that my kundalini awakening began in 2003. I realize now that this was when the first, undeniable expressions of the energy began.

I was never the healthiest of children. I wasn't necessarily sickly, and I could do things like play basketball, but I was plagued by digestive issues and headaches that turned into migraines when I was a teenager. I can now recognize this as a part of my pre-kundalini awakening; during a migraine the entire right side of my body would seize up and contract, signifying an awakening of pingala-related energies.

When I was a teenager and in much of college I numbed my sensitivities through varying substances, and so the experience of significant dreams and other spiritual happenings that were beginning to emerge more readily were drowned out. It was at this time that my sensitivities began increasing. I can now look at this period and see how unskilled I was as someone who is sensitive, and how my own internal teenage chaos was magnified by my sponge-like nature which took on the experiences and energies of my classmates.

In my final year of college I put my attention towards graduating and found that since many of my friends at that time had previously graduated, and I was no longer living in a house that was filled with the clouds and fumes of a continual party, the fog began clearing from my mind. During college I met many people who were in a continual haze, and although we got along reasonably well, if I had known myself better I would not have chosen to live in a house that had six other people living there, as I did not understand things like that I need a certain amount of solitude, or at the very least to not be in a house that was continually chaotic, to not be in a state of nervous system overwhelm.

During this period of time I began changing. I didn't think much about this because I knew that I was going through the expected initiations of adulthood: finding out who I might be, where I might work, graduating from college, and getting married. But I also began to do things that were directed by some inner intuition and urgency.

At age fifteen I picked up a book on Zen Buddhist meditation and a copy of Israel Regardie's *The Middle Pillar* and began meditating, but this was about as regular of a practice as my attempts at working with Llewelyn-style books about herbalism and varying occult practices. I had the books and read them, but didn't engage with the practices consistently enough to get anywhere. I now recognize in myself (and others who are at this stage) that I simply wasn't ready to.

Around the age of twenty I started meditating on a daily basis, picked up pamphlets for yoga and Reiki courses, and engaged again, more seriously, in hermetic as well as other occult traditions. My mailbox filled with pamphlets for Chinese medicine and massage schools that I could only vaguely recall asking for. In my conscious mind, I was still not really processing what I was doing, but I can recognize now that I was basically setting myself up for what was to come.

During this time I found myself experiencing energy surges throughout my body and feeling twitches in varying muscles. I thought little about it until I was twenty-three, when I began doing spontaneous backbends and feeling massive waves of energy like lightning exploding through me on a regular basis.

The First Wave of Kundalini

I began an energy work practice at age twenty-three, and over the next decade I felt that small push that I first felt in my early twenties turn into a massive force of energy that propelled me towards a Master's degree in Chinese medicine, certifications in massage therapy, Asian Bodywork Therapy, two forms of CranioSacral therapy, Zero Balancing, many forms of Reiki, and so many workshops that I have lost count. At one point I was enrolled full time in a four-year graduate degree (Chinese medicine), self-employed seeing 10–20 clients a week, an instructor for the Massage/Asian Bodywork school I had graduated from, and traveling or taking upwards of ten workshops a year, as well as going through a kundalini awakening that drastically changed my consciousness and created severe physical symptoms.

Even looking at this list now, or leafing through my binder of varying certifications, degrees, and workshop certificates, has me a bit dumbfounded about how I accomplished all of this within a decade. It is hard to describe how kundalini flowing through you can be such a profound catalyst, or how it is possible to be physically quite exhausted and spiritually have a large amount of energy.

Although I had been interested in psychology and the occult since I was fairly young, my interest in spiritual healing, magic and folk traditions, and many different forms of religious and spiritual paths exploded during this decade, and I began practicing various ritual and magical works regularly. Although the purpose of magical ritual can be described as a lot of things, depending on the path, what it ultimately does is shift your reality. It does this sometimes quite drastically.

When I began experiencing kundalini with symptoms dramatic enough for me to not deny or repress them, I found a group online that was supportive of people going through kundalini experiences, and it helped me first begin to realize what I was going through, and to get an initial framework that was essential to me making sense of a process like this. I am still very thankful for Bob, as well as the yogis and others online who gave me initial instruction, books to read, and the realization that I was not alone with my experiences.

During this decade of my life I experienced a wide range of changes and symptoms, but the most difficult ones were primarily physical. My digestive system got to the point where I could eat only rice and avocados for six months to a year at a time. I experienced a small tightening of the paraspinal muscles (the muscles next to the spine) as well as electrical sensations in my spine continually. While sometimes this was painful, more often it was like hearing a clock tick in a room in which there was no clock. Symptoms like these were a continual reminder that the process I was undergoing was not simply a psychic upheaval of identity or release of old trauma, but that it was a rewiring process, a process that rebalances and deeply disrupts the neuro-endocrine systems of the body. It was a letting go of what stood in the way of greater realization, consciousness, and enlightenment through the human form.

I would regularly have experiences of a sort of bright light emerging in my chest or head, and then thirty seconds later some aspect of myself, or the world, that I really had thought was true, I now knew to be illusion. I began having increasing dreams and visions that brought forward insights and deeper spiritual experiences. Such experiences were disorienting, and I often needed additional education as well as time to understand and integrate them.

Although I have always been something of a voracious reader, I read countless books until 2008, when I had a near-death experience that left me unable to read or really process very much for about a year.

My menstrual cycles were frequently difficult during this period of time, with energy shooting up through my spine to the top of my head, often with vomiting or nausea involved. I would lie in my bed for hours, feeling waves of processing trauma flow through me, old emotions and experiences coming up in me that often made no sense. At the start of one of my menstrual cycles, I experienced a volcanic force surging up through my midline, flowing up and through my crown. I began vomiting and didn't stop for twenty-four hours, long beyond the time that I had anything in my system left to purge. I was checked into the hospital, given fluids and sent home. When my body was still attempting to throw up a day later, and I realized the likelihood of my death on many different levels, I went back to the hospital.

I checked out of the hospital a few days later against medical advice. I am grateful for the antiemetics (combined with a sedative, so I had little recall of the days I was in the hospital) that saved my life, but doctors could not tell me what had happened to me. Even though I understood that such an experience was spiritual, I still very much wanted some sort of concrete scientific understanding. In this I hoped that it could be prevented from happening again, and to have control over such a possibility.

Initially I went to a near-death support group but found that it was filled with people who were curious about general spiritual topics but had not had a near-death experience, or with people who had an entirely positive experience with the matter. I felt displaced by the fact that many of them were fixated on such an experience and constantly wanted to say how wonderful and special they were for having it. All I wanted to know was how to live after such a profound shift.

The strangest symptom I experienced after my near-death experience was a feeling as if my physical body were an ill-fitting suit—a feeling of being somehow larger than my body and sensing the places where my shoulder was scrunched, where my body felt constrained and blocked. My whole body would vibrate and I felt so much larger and lighter than the physical form I occupied.

This feeling dissipated over time, and I recognize now that many of my initial experiences were a massive purge of emotions that were holding me back, specifically the primary fear we all hold in regards to death. I also recognize now the massive amount of energy that had been flowing through me that had directed me to endless workshops, four years of Chinese medicine school (I was in my last year of a four year program of study at the time of my near-death experience), and rather obsessive study as well as attempts to hold down a full-time job severely depleted me, and led to my nervous system being unable to contend with it all.

For many years I denied that it was a near-death experience because I did not technically die; yet I had many of the same symptoms and experiences as those that I read about. The profound effect that such an experience had on my life was not reconciled until many years later, thanks to exceptional support from bodyworkers and other healers. Later, when I studied tantra and other esoteric systems that work with a body-based approach to enlightenment, I began to make greater sense of the connection between the menstrual cycle, my near-death experience, and the rising of kundalini.

Even today I experience a surge in kundalini and greater creative capacity with my menstrual cycle. It is a profound time of reflection, of meditation, and of connecting; connecting to the power of the creative principle has allowed for me to be deeply rooted in the feminine instead of denying or repressing it.

The Pause In Between

I jokingly say that a lot of my spiritual path was led by the fact that I could always tell when people were lying, or when circumstances were not right. When I was younger I lacked the nuance to understand why people were lying, and that many people are not consciously aware that they are lying.

My capacity to spot what lacked truth or authenticity has likely led me as far on my spiritual path as any other trait. Other people typically extol more spiritual factors such as meditative or past-life spiritual efforts for why they have experienced a significant spiritual calling in their lifetime. I had a type of curiosity that hungered for truth. For many years my spiritual path was led by the seeking of *truth*, and I discovered that whatever depths I reached, there was always yet deeper terrain to explore.

The laughable difficulty about this is that it is a never-ending loop: when I figured out some aspect of myself or the Universe or a particular area of study, my sensitivities increased as a result of that study. This meant that yet again I was in a place of needing to figure out what was going on with myself.

I now approach this with curiosity, rather than frustration or obsession. Being willing to see the falseness at each level, along with being willing to see the falseness or ego within myself, has allowed me to move forward on a path that it is so easy to stagnate on.

It took me a long time to understand that knowledge has layers. At a certain point beyond words knowledge gives way; there is no real neat and tidy truth to be found. The more I explore, the more I see the futility of my initial efforts to find a singular truth—one that lines up with all of the other spiritual truths and frameworks and dogmas. Truth is too large, too magnificent. What we can do is point to the truth in our own way, get out of the way of our ego that is always seeking to be superior or more advanced than we are, and to do the best we can at providing language for the ineffable.

It took me much of that first decade to let go of that need for truth, and to stop myself from mentally latching on to my spiritual experiences. I have learned that reducing such experiences to mental knowings causes them to take on aspects of un-truth, which is something I contend with as a writer on a daily basis.

I continued with my obsessive search for truth and understanding until 2013, ten years after the energy first erupted. By 2011, I had found that my enthusiasm for outward study was waning, and though I had quit traveling to find spiritual teachers and gurus, I was taking local workshops out of habit. One day in 2013 I found myself sitting in yet another workshop and realized that I didn't need to be there. I no longer needed to prove myself to the outer world, I no longer needed to accumulate more initials to feel worthy. But in this instant in 2013 I realized my most profound education came from my meditation practice and direct spiritual revelation; I had disregarded my own gnosis and spiritual connections even though they far exceeded the depth any of these workshops or physical teachers because they were not a piece of paper that I could show others to prove my worth.

I would much rather be sitting home with my family or connecting directly to nature than be in another classroom; sitting alone in simple silence was cheaper, as well as more profound, than what that teacher had to offer. I realized that what I wanted out of my life was joy, and peace, and that many of these workshops are for people at a different place than what I was emerging into.

This was something I had been considering, but in the course it was like an irrevocable moment, a distinct perspective shift that happens in the spiritual awakening process. I had a sense of myself participating in the noise and chaos of the workshop, and then a greater perspective where I felt still, quiet, and observing. Ramana Maharshi best describes this sort of perceptual shift as going from associating oneself as an actor or character on a screen, to realizing that one is the projectionist or the projection itself.

This is when my path turned from centering around the word *truth* to the word *peace*. It was not as if I no longer had any interest in truth, but that the wounding surrounding the word vanished, and what I truly desired after so many years of struggle was to feel at peace.

In 2013 my kundalini awakening subsided. The focus of my life drastically changed from being primarily about spiritual matters, and educating myself and healing myself through this process, to a quieter, more peaceful state of being that included greater attention to family, friends, and connecting to nature and the outer world.

My attention was brought to how important embodiment is, and the importance of cultivating the physical body, including healing my nervous system. My focus shifted from techniques and education to sitting in silence, to communion, to states of interbeing and connection, similar to what I had found as a child sitting by the birch trees and small lake in my backyard in Minnesota. During this period I also realized how short our time in our physical forms are, how precious our human connections are, and how in our human forms we are meant to connect. I began my first book, *The Spiritual Awakening Guide*, and increased my work with clients who were going through kundalini awakenings.

I first started working professionally as an energy worker in 2003, and quickly added on other modalities, degrees and certifications. I soon found that, despite what I put on my sign or website, people were drawn to me who were sensitive or psychic, who needed spiritual assistance, or who were going through spiritual awakenings. This number increased the more I understood what was going on with my own path, and the more experience I gained in working with people in a spiritual capacity. The greater depths that I have traversed, the greater ability I have had to assist others.

The Second Wave of Kundalini

In 2016, kundalini moved from the background to the forefront of my life again. This was like a second wave of kundalini energy. This time it was not the drastic upheaval or purification process that it was before, but instead a process of gaining peace, stillness, and witnessing of light moving through my system. Instead of energy flowing upward I experienced energy flowing down into my heart area. There was also a directionless flow along with a sense of kundalini periodically working on specific aspects of my body.

I experience my body as flow; areas within me that do not have this type of flow point to areas of static consciousness, to held trauma that can be released. I work in conjunction with this flow to become more self-realized, and find that such a flow is like a creative fount of energy, allowing me to fulfill my childhood wish of becoming an author and allowing me to feel aligned with something and nurtured by something much larger than myself.

Through this alignment kundalini expresses much differently than it used to. Instead of shaking and trauma processing, I find myself going into static postures, ecstatic dancing, or simply sitting quietly while what still needs to be resolved within me emerges. A growing sense of embodiment and truly living in a body that is vitally conscious grows within me.

Focusing on my humanity, on deep feeling, and on accepting my humanness has assisted me much more than focusing on anything of a transcendental nature. I am uncertain if enlightenment can be fully experienced on a permanent basis in the human form, or one that is still immersed in the world.

Through this period I continually heard two things: the first was a shift from my search being about *truth* to being about *peace*. The word "peace" now led my spiritual path, and at times I felt a stillness that was incredibly profound. I sorely missed it when it dissipated. I also began hearing the phrase "let go and let god" continually. I had grown up thinking of the concept of god as a patriarchal one; I saw people who were quite unhealed espousing beliefs regarding God that amounted to hatred and the same superiority complexes that I saw in the "spiritual but not religious" crowd. So I resisted the idea of surrender to such a concept. What I learned from allowing myself to listen to and experience this phrase was a deeper level of surrender, which stopped much of the resistance I felt towards the spiritual path. It also helped me release my anger and grief towards experiencing something like this in the modern world.

For many years I sensed my own darkness, my own Otherness, and the many ways in which I am an outlier in this world. I thought that this was what was wrong with me. It took me a long time to recognize that this is what I have to bring to this world.

Trauma and Otherness

I can now see that I have always been Other, aware of the spiritual layers and depths of reality. It has been a large part of my personal path to accept my experiences, my Otherness, and to work through the trauma and misunderstanding of such experiences: to accept who I am, as well as be willing to offer myself to the outer world.

It wasn't until adulthood that I understood that I was someone that inhabited liminal space in this world. In simple archetypal terms, I am an Outlier. In more complex terms, I was someone who always deeply felt and perceived and for many years didn't understand why others could not meet me at those depths. It took a great deal of healing for me to understand that it wasn't that people didn't want to meet me at those depths, but they lacked the capacity or tools to do so.

I discovered other people who traversed similar depths in my early to mid-twenties. At that time a friend told me that I was simply on a different wavelength from most other people, and due to this people either ignore me, become irritated because I am saying things that do not fit in with their ideologies, or resonate with me (or at the very least are open enough to hear from a different point of view). This was immensely helpful for me and it is a speech I now give to the Others who have come my way in my practice.

It is easy to romanticize or idealize this type of Otherness, or to misconstrue it for the isolating effects of trauma, but it is an incredibly bewildering and often quite painful experience to be Other in this world, even when it is seen clearly for what it is. Such individuals are rarely well met by the world, or even spiritual communities, which ironically can have rather rigid mentalities that decry anyone stepping outside of them.

Those who have been Othered by society or who have experienced trauma often have more natural aptitude to traverse liminal spaces. There are many people who feel Othered by the world, separate because they've experienced trauma or because they feel they are not validated by this world. While this can result in spiritual awakening, the Otherness that I describe here is more of a concept of "sitting on another branch of a tree."

This is a Siberian saying for those who traverse liminal spaces and have the aptitude to navigate the spiritual layers of reality. It results in a high level of connectivity and a perspective and way of being that is quite different than much of society.

However, trauma is a path to awakening. Those who have experienced trauma are often psychically "cracked open," resulting in increased psychic sensitivities, shamanic and spiritual capabilities, and perceptual changes. Awakening due to trauma does not mean that such a person is seeing things clearly, in a balanced manner, or is navigating beyond the space of their own psychological projections, though. Trauma creates disconnection; it requires healing before we can utilize any of the perceptual shifts or capacities that have occurred as a result of it. Awakening requires being grounded and stabilized within the human form. Without that grounding it is easy to create disconnected mythic realities out of trauma. Such a person does not awaken, but is held captive by the contents and creations of their wounded psyche.

Through healing my own early childhood trauma and seeing many sensitive and psychic clients during my kundalini awakening I learned that some of my psychic capacities were a natural evolution of biological instinct. Due to my very early years being in a household of fear and violence, I learned to project my energy forward onto other people to be able to read them and to assess them for danger. I took responsibility for any difficulty they may be having to ensure my own safety.

I was giving a lot of my energy away to people and they could then decide how much they were going to give back to me, the difficulty being that most people were so traumatized that they did not give anything back. I was allowing others to define how I related to them. This was exhausting. At a certain point I had to reconcile that I had created a career out of seeing the darkness in people, to see their trauma and what they held within. Once I learned how to set boundaries, I began to relate to people more clearly. Now I am able to see the goodness or potential in people, although I do admittedly still see the trauma first.

The skills that are required for anyone of high perceptual capacities to live in the world are described in my book, *Managing Psychic Abilities*. I do also suggest skilled bodywork, such as CranioSacral therapy, to help to rewire and re-educate the nervous system. Because our nervous system and ways of energetic relating are developed when we are quite young, we end up mirroring the systems of our primary caregivers, and having a system reflective of our childhood environment. Often we do not realize that we can recalibrate this system, and the importance of doing so in any system that was not given the safety, care and attention it deserved in early childhood.

Reconciling my Otherness has ironically made me more of an outlier in many ways in this world; by traversing deeper paths in Spiritual, religious, and occult studies I find myself far beyond what the typical mainstream discourse is on those things.

It also allowed for me to separate what is dark from what is traumatized within me. I can now embody the power held within my atavistic instincts, and understand that the healing of my darkness comes through grounding in these instincts, rather than repressing or denying them. I can now welcome with compassion any aspect of myself that has separated due to trauma. It has been through ecstatic dance, through trauma healing, through meditation and bodywork, that kundalini has allowed me to see both my Otherness and my otherness as simply who I am. They are my divine potential that I bring into the world, and allow me to be of service in a way I could not be without them.

A Path of Service

I am still growing into being able to see clearly that for a decade of my life I devoted myself to little else but my spiritual path: educating myself, studying, experiencing, and immersively exploring. Propelled by kundalini awakening, that period of my life truly was intensive and demanding.

It is hard to describe even fifteen years after that first eruption how much denial I went through with regard to what I was experiencing, how much fear and anger. Along with bringing up massive amounts of latent, body-held trauma for me to acknowledge and resolve, the process was traumatizing in and of itself. It wasn't until I was thirty years old that I even mentioned to anyone that I was experiencing a kundalini awakening. Until that time I did find support online, which got me through an incredibly difficult time in my life. I didn't mention any of it out loud to family or friends until much later and I still don't discuss it much in my private life, as I don't particularly feel the need.

It is also something of an irony that once I got comfortable enough knowing that I was experiencing a kundalini awakening, the label and my fear of it vanished. The process of kundalini awakening is incredibly difficult, but many of my initial experiences were heightened or exacerbated because

I wasn't giving them proper regard. At one point I realized that a percentage of my symptoms and initiatory experiences along this path were due to my disbelief. I saw that I needed to *work with kundalini*, rather than view it as something antagonistic within me. I began to look at it as a privilege; despite a lot of pain and difficulty it was bestowing upon me glimpses of grace, ecstatic states, and expansion of consciousness.

While some of the blissful states and other transcendental states are incredible, we should not stagnate in them. The creative force that flows through someone who has awakened kundalini, the light that shines from them, if they manage to not get stuck in the trauma and ego-aspects of the process, can bring so much to the world. I am able to write, paint, teach, and create quite quickly when I am in a state of flow, in which I am indeed working with kundalini, and for that I have an immense amount of gratitude. It is in this flow state that I feel totally liberated, completely free, and able to recognize and fulfill my divine potential.

I have had symptoms disappear that I thought I would have to live with forever. This does not mean that I am in perfect health, or perfect bliss, but in a continual state of evolution that I both deeply value and still struggle with. Evolution creates change, and change is always difficult. What happens with the spiritual path is that what is not working in your life makes itself very evident or falls away. This can be quite painful, whether it results in or arises from expanded consciousness, ecstatic states, and moving beyond personal limitations.

Our world is in desperate need of lightworkers—ones not stuck in the clouds, but who have traversed their very depths, who are grounded in this world and in their adult capacity to meet the world as it is, who have healed their trauma, and who have decided to work with processes like these with dedicated effort. It is so easy to be led to outer authorities, to illusory wisdom. Those who are willing to look within and take responsibility for themselves are in desperately short supply.

The healing path, the path of acceptance, is really about learning to meet the world. I find that most of mainstream spirituality disconnects people, and gives them illusions that they should separate themselves in a bubble. That perpetuates the cycle of pain, the unhealed tendencies of people not yet awakened enough to realize that the world is how it is and people are who they are. Being grounded in the world means meeting others with clarity instead of expecting them to adhere to our personal ideologies. Instead of spiritual awakening being something that isolates me, I can connect better and find a part of myself that resonates with each person that I meet. The enlightenment process does not happen outside of the body. The human form and its senses should be celebrated, and it is by connecting deeply to our emotions, to our senses, and to our innate humanness that we can truly love and accept ourselves, as well as experience joy in our lives, in the short time that we are in human bodies.

As of this writing I am in a state of feeling a downward flow into my heart area. The rise of kundalini goes into my head and brain where it is still experiencing restrictions. I witness myself becoming more and more embodied, less reactive to the outer world, more compassionate, and have much stronger boundaries than I used to. I look to people, places, and things in this world that I feel disconnected from, or that I cannot look compassionately towards, as the areas that could use healing work within me.

I am grounded in my life again, and realize how fleeting it is to be within the human form. How precious our connections are to one another, how quickly they pass. I am much more aware of the passage of time, and acutely aware of how I spend my time.

I am deeply aware that the first part of the spiritual path for anyone must fixate on the self. It is a healing and purification process to gain greater perspective. But beyond that phase, a deepening awareness of how you can be of service to the world and what you bring to the world develops. The realization that the spiritual path is not one of self-obsession, but that you are healing yourself, your family, your community, and the world in some small way through awakening. It is by realizing the spark of the divine in you that you can spark another.

People who are undergoing awakenings of any kind have the ability to do this, to spark others, and are very much needed in this day and age to assist a world that is so filled with trauma, that so lacks remembering on any conscious level of what it is like to be connected to anything. The spiritual path requires effort, it requires knowledge, and is one of the most difficult things that anyone can do. I applaud anyone willing to consciously walk it, to heal, to awaken.

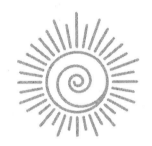

2

The Nature
of Kundalini

The experience of kundalini awakening through the midline of the body brings about a revolutionary, evolutionary process. We move from having little to no conscious awareness of anything beyond ourselves and our own immediate needs to knowing and embodying our true potential in this world.

Consider the perspective of looking out at the universe through a peephole. This is an *asleep* state, in which we look out at the world through a very narrow perspective—what we personally know, have directly experienced, or have been taught by family and society to be valid. As we awaken, the peephole widens. We begin to see other perspectives, to understand the forces and traumas that have created us. We release what has constricted the peephole: the traumas, experiences, and ideologies that have shaped our world and identity.

The more we release, the more the peephole widens. We become more conscious, our perspective changes. We begin to realize what is beyond that peephole, and to extricate ourselves from the traumas and social conditionings that have stopped us from experiencing self-realization. We begin to interface directly with spiritual energy and the dynamic nature of consciousness itself. We begin to really see the world for what it is, rather than what we would like for it to be, and to let go of needing others to act in accordance to our personal ideologies. Kundalini awakening is the activation of the spiritual power that lies latent within our systems. This energy is at the base of our spine within our sacrum, and when activated, it emerges and uncoils through the spinal column and head. Through this uncoiling, our consciousness expands and we evolve spiritually, physically, and emotionally.

Kundalini as Consciousness

If we look at understandings of the cosmos that offer the perspective that everything is consciousness, such as forms of Buddhism and Kashmir Shaivism, we can view kundalini as consciousness and potential that lies within our human form. When kundalini awakens, it unfolds and rises within us, and we become increasingly conscious, expanding beyond basic self-interest into a greater perspective.

One of the paradoxes of kundalini awakening is that it is simultaneously an expansion process that brings greater perspective and the ability to access cosmic consciousness, as well as a contracting or individuating process that allows us to realize our individual potential as human beings.

Within our midline, we have an *axis mundi*, a world tree, a spiritual highway that allows for our consciousness to unfold. When kundalini rises up this axis mundi, going from the roots of the tree (in the genitals and sacrum area), to the very tips of the branches (the crown and above the head), we complete the first two stages of kundalini awakening. The experience of rainfall (grace) flowing through the branches to reach the roots, as well as fully flowing through the trunk (the "heart" of the tree) is the last stage of kundalini awakening and brings permanent realization.

When we awaken it may just be an initial flow from root to branch; it may also be a permanently unfolding process that allows for full realization. The tree within us truly thrives when the flow goes from root to branch, from earth to root, as well as from sky to branch, and branch to trunk. Understanding this can allow for a shift away from misunderstandings about the process. In simpler terms, one rainstorm from the sky or one experience of flow from the roots upwards is very different from the tree flowing permanently and continuously.

In other perspectives, kundalini is Shakti, or the power of spiritual manifestation, creativity, sexuality, and power. It is the dynamic energy of creation that is the basis of life and existence. In the process of a kundalini awakening this dynamic, feminine creative principle rises to meet the static, male principle known as Shiva, which is located above the crown. This is the pathway of individual consciousness meeting cosmic or universal consciousness. It is the energy of the female pole ascending and meeting the male pole, the two principles that hold us in polarity and trap us in illusion and limited perspective. After male and female poles have merged, the undifferentiated creation energy can then flow through us.

If we look at the state of the world, it is no wonder that we revere the masculine state of stillness and emptiness, while disregarding the feminine powers of creation and evolution. We live in a patriarchal society that has suppressed and denied the feminine power of creation. Our bodies, the spirit world, the natural world, and our emotions are the deep feminine wisdom within us. These have all been taken away, destroyed, or demonized.

The masculine pole places us within binary consciousness. In somatic studies it is represented by the head, the energy of "doing," and our logical minds. We need this force to bring our ideas into light, to act on our feminine intuition. In masculine types of consciousness, two polarities will always be at odds with one another. The masculine vs. the feminine, me vs. someone else—what we view as opposite and warring forces within and without.

Consciousness rooted in the feminine pole has a triple form: the power to see two things but also what lies between them, to access liminal space, to continually create and re-create. Ultimately this is the power we all emerge from to separate into binary consciousness. It is only by deeply revering the feminine power of creation, by connecting the head to the body, the masculine to the feminine, that we can move beyond the constructs of binary reality and into a recognition of the creative principle that birthed us all.

It is an incorrect assumption to state that kundalini awakening is purely feminine, or goddess energy. It certainly never stops being the power of creation and evolution, which are deeply feminine powers. But enlightenment comes as the masculine and feminine forces within us intertwine and support instead of opposing one another. By merging these principles of feminine and masculine, we move beyond a state of separation into wholeness and thus become fully realized. We become female and male, empty and full. We can even go beyond those states to witnessing them, witnessing consciousness or the tides of energy flowing through our system.

In kundalini awakenings the state of completion is not one of a simple circuit of energy flowing from the genitals through the top of the head or into the brain, but of both forces combining and becoming one, and both flowing downward, intertwined, into the heart space. This is a state of being beyond two forces constantly at odds with one another within and without—male and female, void and non-void, expansion and contraction, fullness and emptiness. This is a state of being both forces simultaneously, as well as dropping between them.

The separation of these two forces creates the duality of this world. The rising of kundalini from the genitals through the spinal column to the brain is the interplay or dance of these two forces, with the eventual result being a "marriage" in which the two forces are no longer viewed, felt, or understood as separate.

Kundalini is responsible for our very creation, for everything contained within our reality. It is consciousness, the basic building block of our reality. It is responsible for our physical form, for our physiological processes like digestion. As this energy folds and differentiates, it becomes less clear, less powerful, and we step further away from our original energy. We become more and more steeped in illusion, anchored to the folds and differentiations, rather than understanding our authentic nature.

Kundalini and Qi

One of the most difficult things to understand is the paradox of kundalini energy. It both creates everything and yet is described as being a latent force. We are all part of the dynamic unfolding of kundalini. We all breathe, have spirit, live our lives. We all have energy (or qi), which is the differentiated or "folded" force that moves through our body and which can be cultivated by practices like martial arts, yoga, meditation, and energy work. The cultivation of our energy is an important discipline; many of us interested in a spiritual path explore a variety of modalities and disciplines in order to understand, feel, and work with our energy.

It is a part of the kundalini awakening process that our qi opens up our meridians (the channels and pathways of the body) in preparation for the flow of kundalini energy. However, it is easy to confuse this preparatory process for kundalini awakening itself. But qi can be described as a differentiated stream as opposed to the deeper, more massive force that is kundalini. Or a separated creek as opposed to the vast, cosmic ocean where that creek originates.

Many people involved in spiritual pursuits feel the differentiated energy of qi flowing through their systems and assume that it is kundalini. The difference between feeling differentiated energy and feeling the primal, atavistic power that is kundalini is like the difference between a babbling brook and a massive tsunami; between a single wave and the oceanic depths.

Both types of awakening are important; we awaken to spirit in many different ways. Differentiated qi is responsible for maintaining our human forms and lives as well as the life of everything on earth. The experience of qi can bring great healing and awareness; it can also indicate pre-kundalini states.

An Overview of Kundalini Awakening

During a kundalini awakening we move from feeling as if we are human beings experiencing something spiritual to a direct experience of our transcendent nature. We move from being someone who feels like kundalini is increasing our consciousness to understanding that kundalini is consciousness and that we are consciousness. We can even move into a state beyond that of witnessing consciousness itself.

As the snake of kundalini unfolds within and up our midlines, we move from basic self-interest into greater awareness. Each time that the snake uncurls we move to a new stage of being. Each chakra or knot that we move through is an initiatory process in which our individual consciousness evolves. With the first uncurling of the snake, we are focused on self-healing. This is the arousal of the first and second chakras, located in the genitals and lower abdomen. In this stage, the focus is still on the self. We begin to realize that we are more than the chaos and noise that makes up our daily lives.

While the entirety of kundalini awakening can be called a purification process, during the first stage the focus is often on early childhood and areas that are well covered by modern psychology, as well as the ancestral and past life patterns that have contributed genetically or spiritually to our limited understanding of who we are.

The first phase of kundalini awakening is the fire purification phase—the release of past trauma out of the system. In this stage the fire and heat generated through kundalini awakening burns away our personal and transpersonal traumas.

During the second stage of kundalini awakening, the snake uncurls its second and third aspects, and the focus is on the third chakra (solar plexus) through heart chakra, in which we have made it beyond basic self-interest and are now beginning to look at the world and ourselves with greater perspective.

In this second stage we go from being someone who "has kundalini" to someone who is experiencing kundalini. While this seems like a small distinction, it is the beginning of understanding that the force rising within us is consciousness itself, and that many of our previous experiences were byproducts, or releases of limited perspective, in order to realize the self as consciousness.

During this phase we begin to separate from the unhealed material of our first and second chakras and to resolve many of those patterns. The dramas we enact for ourselves, the illusions, the egoic needs such as being superior to others, dissolve. By seeing ourselves as more than just a separate self, fighting against ourselves, the world, and the people in it, we begin to understand and feel compassion for those around us.

As solar plexus and heart chakras are pierced by the snake rising within, we realize that what we see in the outer world is a projection. In tantric understanding each person that we run across is an aspect of ourselves, and we can look inward to resolve what we react to in the outer world. In other systems this is called "shadow work." In this phase we experience the basic underlying connection between ourselves and others. We begin to recognize oneness as more than an intellectual concept. A perspective shift occurs: we see that we can utilize the outer world, the people in it, and any personal suffering that remains, to understand what is blocking further realization.

This is a deconditioning process, which allows us to heal remaining persecutor issues (the times that we, our ancestors, or past lives, have created harm in this world). We extricate ourselves from enmeshment with what society, culture, or the world seeks for us to do or to be.

As the snake unfolds its third curl, kundalini makes its way through the throat and into the third eye. At this stage we begin to realize that we *are* consciousness. As kundalini moves into the brain, we experience immense light as well as an indescribable sensation of flow. We are a drop in the ocean of divine consciousness and at the same time the entirety of that ocean. This can feel quite blissful; it is referred to as en-light-enment for a reason. We experience clear light, grace, ecstatic states, and tremendous flow through the body. In this stage we begin to do internal work for the benefit of the world and the people in it; we surrender to divine grace and are led by it.

In the final stage the last half curl of the snake unfolds from the third eye through the crown. The snake has straightened its three and a half curls and kundalini can permanently flow through the midline and throughout the body. This is commonly referred to as ego death, in which we experience being one with the Universe, undifferentiated, part of the totality instead of merely an individualized human in a physical form. The fear of death dissolves. A drastic reorganization process occurs in which we no longer focus on the sort of commotion and projections emerging out of trauma and blind emotive reaction, nor identify with the human form as the dominant force and concern in our existence.

After the crown has fully opened, the feminine and masculine energies of the body can move permanently into wholeness. Once this has occurred, the now undifferentiated force can flow back downward, opening the spiritual heart and completing the process of enlightenment.

Some choose to postpone achieving full enlightenment in order to be of service to their fellow humans, to be a catalyst or assistant for the evolution of humankind. This is the path of the Bodhisattva. There is an old Zen saying that many of you probably know: "Before enlightenment chop wood and carry water; after enlightenment, chop wood and carry water." The end of the path is the descent of grace—a return to the human form with a feeling of flow and penetration through the heart.

In any type of grounded spirituality, which does not reject the importance of the human form, the eventual result of awakening is to bring oneself back to the world and to experience enlightenment through the physical form. From Plato's *Allegory of the Cave* to Zen realizations of enlightenment, the completion of the path is expressed as clarity that we carry into our daily activities, letting go of attachment and being of service.

An activity that is meant to transcend the body or its senses is temporary, and for a distinct purpose: to shift the perspective of the body and its consciousness. In later phases of awakening there is a reintegration with the senses and the physical form, but without being hooked into them as we were in less conscious states.

We often grasp onto transcendental states, as we do many spiritual experiences, to use them to fuel personal ideologies, rather than to experience liberation. While experiences of emptiness, bliss, love, or ecstasy are important, what is happening in such states is often the creation of a road map. It is much easier to travel down a new road with a map than without one. While experiences of kundalini temporarily arising can be quite spectacular, it is easy to mistake the creation of a road map with permanent attainment.

Challenges along the Path

It is hard to describe to those wholly invested in the spiritual path that at a certain point the obsessive and all-encompassing nature of the path gives way to utter simplicity. We attend to the human form and realize how precious life is, how we are meant to connect. With the descent of grace, we work through what is preventing us from connecting to ourselves, one another, and the world. Clear light and the sensation of flow are felt throughout the body, and the areas of static consciousness continue to resolve. When the senses open, emotions can flow, and we can deeply and authentically feel. Our attention turns beyond personal selfishness to others in this world, communing through our senses, allowing deep acceptance of everything, both inside and outside of ourselves.

In the early stages we are so traumatized and caught in our own chaos that we create the illusion that by healing ourselves we will get to some inhuman state of no longer feeling, or experiencing only love. Yet it is paradoxically by deeply feeling, by opening the senses wide, by accepting all of our emotions as valid, that we can feel love.

Continual effort is required by those who wish to remain in anything beyond the most superficial states of realization. The path of substantial awakening is one of discipline. To have consciousness flow through us on a continual basis requires balance and stability, as well as spiritual, emotional, mental, and physical health.

It is a paradox of this path that a process of moving us into oneness is also a deeply individuating process. Although we are all consciousness, we have different histories, different expressions of the elements within us, different aptitudes in this world. The creativity inherent in kundalini expresses itself in each individual differently—our cycles of birth and death, our physical reproductive capacities, our sexual essence, our ability to create and evolve on so many different levels. Through this process there is realization of our individual divine potential, and the removal through purification of anything that blocks that potential.

Romanticizing this as becoming a great spiritual teacher or a millionaire is the result of illusion. One of the most awakened human beings I know is a high school mathematics teacher. His potential is to use his awakening to reach the students that pass through his school. He is not well paid or famous, but he has very much taken the vow of the Bodhisattva, and has in many ways completed his spiritual path. Many other individuals I know who have attained great consciousness simply return to their daily lives; they live in the joy of deepening connection to themselves and others while they still have the benefit of being in the human form.

Many great artists—painters, thinkers, inventors, musicians, poets— whose creations have emerged from kundalini arising, were not met well in this world, at least during their human lives. Those who walk a profound spiritual path find their lives filled with unique difficulties, which differ from the typical chaos and projections that most people deal with.

The completion of the journey of kundalini awakening is the rise of energy through the midline out of the head and then the descent of grace, flowing on a permanent basis, with clear light emanating through the heart as well as the whole body. But such consciousness can always unfold more clearly, connect more, feel more and flow more. Kundalini is an evolutionary process, and within the human form we can always become more evolved.

Such a path is difficult, and many get lost along the way. There are many traps and illusions along the path. The first is always that we mistake the first step on the spiritual path for the last. The second is that we can so easily immerse ourselves in ungrounded mythic creations rather than integrated or grounded realities. We know when we are steeped in illusion because our mythic versions of ourselves and our everyday reality and inner feelings are too far apart. We always know if something comes from pain or lack of healing. We know when we are wounded, when we are not bringing our authentic selves into the world, when we have put on a mask.

The increased perspective we get as our peephole widens reveals a world filled with illusion, trauma, pain, disconnection, and societal structures that make it impossible for many in our world to truly thrive. This is a painful realization; awareness is not always a gift.

Spiritual flow, or kundalini, arises through our physical forms for a reason. There is no other way for us to evolve; we must transform all aspects of our being, including the dense physical form. It is by looking directly at our projections, at our masks, and at the suffering that is beneath them, that we can awaken.

Expansion and Contraction

The kundalini awakening process is often described as one pole meeting another, thus overcoming duality. However, there is another helpful concept: that of expansion, contraction, and the stillness between such states. While this can be described as the basic birth-death cycle, or the generation-destruction cycle, we can also view expansion and contraction as waves moving outward and inward like tides.

In Chinese medicine, the basic energetics of the human form are that of expanded and contracted states. Our energy field expands—we wish to take in, to be active and dynamic, to engage in study and experiences that expand our understanding of who we are. We are more extroverted, excited, and immersed in the outer world.

In contraction states our energy field moves inward. We digest our prior experiences, we attend to our inner needs and processes. This is a period of self-reflection, of introversion, and of integrating into the personality what was previously absorbed.

Beyond personal energetics, we can look to the expansion and contraction of individual, societal, and cosmic energies. They each have their individual cycles of expansion and contraction, all of which affect us. For many women cycles are easier to notice as menstruation naturally places us in an often obvious pattern. During the first half of our cycle (from day three or five of our cycle) we typically are more expansive, and then mid-way through our cycle (day 14, or when there is ovulation and a shift in hormones) we become more contracted, feeling a deep need for introversion, dreaming, and introspection.

Individually we all experience smaller and larger cycles of contraction and expansion. Expansion feels freeing, it feels exciting, and appropriate in the productivity ethos of our culture. That said, we may stop ourselves in expansion phases, if we are terrified of change or growth that comes with new perspective and greater consciousness. But we are even less comfortable with contraction states that require nurturing, especially nurturing of ourselves, and may have deep wounds, societal constraints, or everyday concerns that prevent us from doing so.

Societally, culturally, and cosmically we also go through states of expansion and contraction. People have described these in different ways throughout the centuries: as a pendulum swinging, as a journey around the wheel of death and birth, as a mythic descent into the Underworld and then an ascent into the Heavens.

The way that I now experience such energies is as a wave. There is the wave that is going back out to sea, and then the wave that is crashing on the shore. Expansion—back to sea. Contraction—back to shore. The more I experience kundalini within my system and the more that it flows through my system unimpeded, the more that I recognize it as a wave form, a flow within me. I am far from the first to have a realization of this, but if we can recognize such cycles we can attend to them, learn to ride them out, utilize them.

Finally, and most powerfully, we can discern a pause, a still point of sorts, between each of the cycles. If our world is created and differentiated at first through duality—feminine and masculine, stillness and dynamism, expansion and contraction—what is in between those states is the undifferentiated ground of original reality. What comes before the folds, what comes before the creation of duality.

It is by sitting at this conjunction, in between the states of contraction and expansion, that we attune to our original nature. This is not a state of emptiness, but paradoxically a state of stillness and dynamism simultaneously. We can realize who we were before the process of differentiation; and in that, we have a glimpse of infinity.

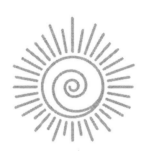

3

The Chakra System and Kundalini

As kundalini awakens, our inner snake rises through the midline, piercing through the chakra system. Although the number of chakras can vary by tradition and system, in this work we will consider that we have seven chakras, which is the number commonly used in modern Western thought.

Our first chakra is located in many individuals at the juncture between our coccyx (the pointy tip of our tailbone) and anus, and flows downward through our perineum, expanding through the genitals and into the earth when open. Our seventh chakra is located at the crown of the head. Kundalini rises and creates a pillar of light going through the midline, straight out the top of the head.

When kundalini flows continuously, it activates centers in the brain as well as the *bindu* point, which is just above and a little behind the crown. This activation allows for greater consciousness, as well as a cycling of energies back down into the brain, heart, and digestive system. The complete activation of the *bindu* point would allow for full conscious control of the nervous system, including the ability to consciously choose the time of death. While the permanent awakening of consciousness is an aspiration for many, the activation of the used *bindu* point is quite rare and does not occur without concerted effort over many decades, or even lifetimes.

Each chakra can be considered a level on an elevator of consciousness. We go from the ground floor (the first chakra) to the top floor (the crown chakra), each floor resulting in an expansion of consciousness. Chakras also can be considered initiatory gateways; this means that a specific type of understanding and release needs to occur so that kundalini can pass through that gateway and continue to flow upwards.

Each time that kundalini unfolds and rises on a permanent basis to a new chakra, we release what was held in the previous chakra and evolve into a greater perspective. If we look at the chakra system, when kundalini is unawakened we are essentially in a state of "sleep." We care little about anything beyond our most immediate needs, we are unable to see perspectives outside of our own, and we have little awareness of how we get hooked into patterns of behavior that emerge out of unhealed trauma. We feel isolated and alone, and may lack compassion. We attend to the dramas and chaos of our existence, not noticing that whatever we are experiencing is often temporary, illusory, or self-created.

The First Chakra

When kundalini awakens in the first chakra, we begin to understand how our past has created who we are. We attend to our basic psychology and make basic connections between our childhood and our wounding patterns. Any type of awakening is still entirely self-serving; we neither notice others nor have much compassion for them. We grasp onto spiritual experiences as a way to create more drama or attention for ourselves; what is unhealed within us creates mythic realities out of any spiritual experience.

For most of us who have awakened kundalini, the first chakra is where we get stuck. We may need such experiences in order to feel superior, or we may become obsessed with the experience itself. We enjoy the drama, even if it is painful drama, as it makes our lives interesting and offers purpose. On some subconscious level we are aware that moving forward would create a perspective shift, but we are not ready for that.

If kundalini has awakened in the first chakra, but is blocked from rising upwards, it can create immense difficulties in the genitals and lower abdomen. This can be experienced as extreme heat in the genital area, heightened sexual feelings that only find release through masturbation or sexual relations, itching in the genitals and thighs (particularly the perineum), and emotional-mental instability. We may become unstable, ungrounded, and dysfunctional in the world but believe that we are somehow highly conscious and evolved. This is exacerbated by the fact that frequently the awakening of kundalini can cause bursts of energy out of the head or in other regions of the body. We can enter incredible states, such as transcendental bliss and emptiness, with even the smallest expression of kundalini awakening in the human form. It is easy to latch on to such experiences. The illusion that comes from having "fire in the head" without a permanent residence of kundalini energy there can immerse us in unhealed realities and divert us from forward progress.

The Second Chakra

The first chakra is an initiatory gate. Passage to the second involves moving beyond basic self-interest to seeing and attending to others in a compassionate way. At first this can be tinged with self-interest; we see our family, our pets, or charities that have had an effect on us, and feel expanded interest and love towards them. This is often through societally based notions of being "good" or what is morally correct. It is when the heart chakra opens that we can fully gain perspective beyond our own self-interest. It is when the third eye opens that we can individuate from societal conditioning.

The second chakra and first often go together; there is a "knot" (discussed later), which is an initiation beyond basic self-interest and involvement. The initiation of the second chakra is the same as the first, in that all of the initiations have to do with the same subject: ego. Our ego is our identity, our mind, and it has a vested interest in us remaining who we think we are. Any change is perceived as danger, as death, and so there is strong resistance to change. Our ego is the sum of our wounds, what is false about us, and it is only by going through multiple processes of "ego death," by dissolving and evolving our identity, that we can discover our cosmic "I"—our true potential in conjunction with divinity.

The first and second chakras express what is important to us, our intimate connections and personal interests. In the second chakra, located in most people midway between the genitals and the belly button, we are likely to have heat and disruption as kundalini emerges. Significant digestive difficulties, gynecological issues, and continued first chakra issues can occur. We become increasingly aware of how family and ancestry, as well as past lives, have affected us.

The Third Chakra

Whereas in the mainstream map of the chakras, the third has to do with the solar plexus (so as to make the chakras "even" on the map), in this model the third chakra involves the digestive system, specifically the small intestine (the area around the belly button).

In the kundalini awakening process, the digestive fire is severely disrupted. We develop an awareness of how foods affect the system, and we can even become unable to process certain foods. This can be quite drastic, such as an inability to eat anything but rice for periods of time, or extreme stomach bloating to the point of looking pregnant. There can also be difficult emotional upheavals, especially if there is a lack of balance emotionally or mentally.

The small intestine is called *the second brain* for a reason. We need a place to hold the emotions that we weren't able to express or even feel throughout our lives. We are a sick culture when it comes to emotions. Heavy social conditioning teaches us to numb any emotions that would be considered negative. Through such cultural norms we try to ignore any "dark" emotions or to control them.

We carry a lot within us that is quite dark and traumatized. Our internal rage does not want to be hugged and offered a puppy. It wants to rage, and to be accepted in that rage. As we awaken the third chakra, we begin to move out from the considerable trauma that has been binding us to a very incomplete, fragmented, and isolated view of the universe. We begin to accept even the very darkest aspects of ourselves.

The initiation in the third chakra is an acceptance of every bit of oneself, from the rage to the joy. Thus a profound shift in the kundalini awakening process takes place. It is no longer about personal trauma, or personal healing, but about moving through that initiatory gateway into greater consciousness and acceptance of the world as it is.

Before this point, we tend to think that the world needs to meet us. We believe that others should share the same beliefs, and we create illusions out our need for superiority and inferiority. We lack the recognition that what we hate outwardly is a result of division within ourselves. We create mythical realities based on what is unhealed within, and participate in a huge amount of noise and commotion because that is what we believe life is.

At this point on the path, we can begin to create conspiracy theories, thus perpetuating unhealed beliefs about the world and the self. This comes from either a lack of significant spiritual experience or as a result of awakened kundalini being diverted to the wrong channel. We have failed to move past the "gate" into greater experience, and might languish for years or decades (if not lifetimes), as a result of not healing inner trauma or stabilizing ourselves mentally-emotionally.

This is why the first stages of the path involve grounding, clarity, and healing of trauma. Otherwise we never progress forward, whether kundalini has awakened or not. A teacher or healer is often required for us to gain perspective. Sometimes I meet people who are severely imbalanced and who believe that they are a great prophet or have experienced a kundalini awakening of huge magnitude. Often what they are experiencing is dissociation and mental-emotional imbalances that could be attended to if they were willing to seek help.

Education is key. I likewise meet individuals who believe that they have had an extraordinary experience, or that they are enlightened or incredibly conscious because of their experiences. If they were to educate themselves, they would find that many of their experiences are quite common, or that there are many stages beyond them.

While I could lament the state of spiritual studies in this world, or how we have split so far from the spirit realms that we believe we do not need to educate ourselves (or may believe we have mastery after very little education), I find that most individuals are unwilling to educate themselves because they would see that they are not very far on their paths. Our ego has a vested interest in us remaining who and what we are, and it will do anything to keep us from evolving.

Typically such individuals will find unhealed or uneducated teachers who support their illusions or they will believe that they can forgo having a teacher altogether. Further evolution will occur only when the individual is ready to contend with what is unhealed and is willing to seek clarity.

The spiritual path requires effort, and the type of clarity that kundalini awakening offers is often a brutal clarity. It is a rare individual who is willing to let go of transcendent or peak experiences and contend with what is within. We always know if we are in pain, even if we deny it; to move beyond the initiatory gateway of the first three chakras requires attending to that pain.

Kundalini is a purifying process. It is a fire within that reveals and resolves the blockages in our system that prevent us from attaining greater consciousness and eventual liberation. But if we hang on to our lack of clarity stemming from ignorance and trauma, we will not be liberated. A spiritual teacher who has authentically walked this path is hard to find in a world steeped in illusion, but there are some. We may not wish to find them, however, as they are likely to point out that we are not as far on the path as we would like to believe.

The Fourth Chakra

The first curl of kundalini ends after the third chakra. In the next intiatory gate we move on to the solar plexus and heart chakra. There we grow beyond our obsessive need for self-healing and we begin to consider the other forces that have created us.

Much of mainstream spirituality is locked in the first stage of development. Only personal material is considered, with a focus on superiority and narcissistic impulses about being "chosen" or "special." Or there may be a desire to heal within in order to accumulate wealth and to emulate what society determines to be "success."

If we progress further, we move beyond the bubble of the spiritual path, and into recognizing the shared humanity between us. We begin to notice the experiences of other people in this world, and societal implications and injustices. We no longer need our personal ideologies and ethics to be understood and enacted by those around us. We also begin to realize that we alone do not create the world, but that we dream the world communally.

When the heart chakra is pierced by the second uncurling of kundalini energy, there is a greater focus and understanding of consciousness itself. The light of compassion begins to shine. We realize that what we are reactive to in the world is what lies unhealed within us. This is true shadow work. By taking personal responsibility for what lies unhealed within us, what separates us from another human being, we begin to witness, understand, and feel compassion for those around us.

I often compare an unhealed person to someone who is drowning. When we are drowning, all of our attention goes into simply surviving. In an unhealed state, we are unable to notice anything but our own needs to stay alive and get through the day. We might be unconscious of the fact that when we are drowning we could pull those who come close to us into a state of instability, or may even cause them to drown as well.

We have all been in such states, and it is necessary to attend to the self during them. We may need to be a bit selfish; it may be the first time that we have decided to do so. Those who are trained and understand such states can gently guide us back to clarity. Taking responsibility for ourselves often means realizing when we need help. When we heal, when kundalini purifies the system, the heaviness of what we carry lessens. This does not mean we have perfect health, or may never be in the position of drowning again, but that there is a measured stability in the system.

When we move beyond our traumas and emotional baggage, either in the kundalini awakening process or as part of a healing path, we find ourselves more balanced. We can recognize and accept support for times when we feel like we're drowning.

A massive shift in perspective occurs when kundalini awakens the upper chakras. The heart is a sort of pivot point between the lower and upper chakras, where we begin to notice, listen to, and perceive much more than our own personal experiences of this world.

We engage willingly on our path. Through the perspective of the heart we understand how freeing it is to release long-standing beliefs. At the same time, seeing how much we struggled as our previous selves can create immense grief.

The Fifth, Sixth, and Seventh Chakras

When kundalini awakens beyond the heart, our perception deepens and we open to psychic capacities. It is through the third eye that we recognize and move away from the noise and chaos of the world. This perspective shift is difficult to describe, but is what I refer to in my book *The Body Deva* as the "tornado of chaos."

This is not a state of disassociation. Disassociation creates a different vantage point, an ability to see outside of oneself, but rather than an evolved perspective, it is one of great pain and disconnection. The spiritual awakening process is one of both expansion and consolidation simultaneously, giving our mind and emotions a solid and grounded container from which to expand. The psychic and physical structures within the body need to be rewired so awakening can occur; without them, we are unable to properly evolve. Without the stability of our bodies as a container for kundalini to awaken, and without healing past trauma so we can achieve a healthy ego-mind, our perspective shifts will not result in clarity, and we are likely to be significantly lost or stuck in our process.

This perspective shift takes us deeply inward, and it is quite easy for people to get stuck at this gate. We lament a world so filled with noise and illusion, and we may come to think of ourselves as superior because we no longer attend to the nonsense and illusion.

We may get stuck in the vacuum that is created by such a state. If we are no longer creating noise and drama for ourselves, we end up with a lot of time on our hands. We may also find ourselves in a bit of an existential crisis because the world does not recognize such things, and we may stagnate in the loss of meaning that emerges as a result of realizing the world is illusory. If we can recognize that we are here for more than just ourselves, and reorient ourselves to being of service to the world, this sense of meaninglessness dissipates. If we can overcome these blocks, the creative impulse of kundalini completes the cycle of ego death by moving through the crown and blossoming into the divine "I."

There are a series of knots between the third eye and the crown. The initiatory gate of moving beyond the third eye and allowing kundalini to flow to the crown involves the release of the ego, but often not in a way that people commonly imagine.

We require a healthy ego-mind, not an absent one. It is through healing trauma and mental-emotional conflicts that our minds can become clearer and we can become healthier. As a result we can recognize who we are as individuals, as well as what we bring into this world. Any ego death is a transformative process in which the ego-mind is reoriented towards health and greater stability. Without the container of the physical form and a healthy ego-mind, the transformative process of spiritual awakening cannot occur properly.

The emerging of kundalini into the crown creates a meeting or marriage between the forces that govern duality. It also creates enlightenment states of emptiness, ego death, peace, and ecstatic bliss. Many consider this to be the end of the spiritual path. It is true that such experiences are quite high realizations.

This raises again the question of temporary states versus permanence. There are many people who believe they are quite enlightened because they have had a temporary experience of bliss or emptiness. They may even experience many states of bliss, or some permanency of the state. However, because they cling to such experiences and fall into the same ego trap that occurs in every single chakra in different ways, there is typically not any greater self-realization.

The Spiritual Heart

Experiences of lack of meaning and complete undifferentiated oneness give way to the final phase of the path: the opening of the spiritual heart. This is the descent of grace, re-individuation with our physical form, grounding in everyday life, and realization of the cosmic "I."

This cosmic "I" is a feeling of complete flow and opening of the spiritual heart. While the heart chakra may have been previously opened, the spiritual heart has different energetic structures to it. In Ramana Maharshi's system, it is located two digits to the right of the physical heart, in the space of the fourth vertebra (the center of the heart and then laterally to the right).

This is an opening of the energetic structures of the heart, which include the aorta (top of the heart), the pericardium (the heart covering), and the "high heart" which is above the heart and associated with the thymus. The activation of this center allows us to recognize that our purpose is enlightenment within the human, physical form, and to be of service to the world through our unique capacities.

The spiritual heart aligns our unique elements and capacities with cosmic intelligence. When we reach the gateway above the head, paradoxes are reconciled; we understand that something can be one thing and its complete opposite at the same time. We know that opposites live together, inform one another, and are often oddly the same thing. We know that awakening occurs at the conjunction of opposites, and that it is through reconciling paradox that we can awaken. It is through being in the liminal space between paradoxes that we can see through binary existence. Without fully grasping this concept, it is impossible to understand that we can experience both oneness and separation, that one in fact creates the other, and that they exist only in conjunction with one another.

We conceive mental constructs through polarity. The idea that the spiritual path is one of *katabasis*—a descent into the depths and darkness of self in order to rise—cannot be understood by those wishing for a spiritual path in which they do not have to dig around in their own dirt. We can hold light only if we traverse our darkness; we can have "no I" only by discovering what our "I" is. Such things will never be grasped by the intellect or supported by false realization.

When the spiritual heart is open, we feel ever greater compassion for the self and creativity and our divine potential can flow through us unimpeded. This showers the world with grace, while clear light flows through every cell in our human form (en-light-enment).

The initiatory process through these chakras is about surrender. We realize that we can always evolve more, be more. We are willing to realize that it is easy to stagnate either in lack of clarity or lack of knowledge, to project what is unhealed within, and to see the first step (or the five hundred and twelfth) on the path as the last.

What is needed for us to proceed on this path is to be willing to take personal responsibility for ourselves, to look within, and to understand that every stage of the spiritual path presents ego traps for us to proclaim illusory superiority or enlightenment, and then to say "no" to such illusions.

4

The Knots and
Chakra Sheaths

Imagine kundalini energy as an ocean. The objective of a kundalini awakening is for the entirety of the ocean to flow up continually through the midline, making a column that extends through the midline, both above the head and through the genitals into the Earth. This is our connection to the Earth as well as to the divine. Then the flow of that ocean can go to other places in the body, including the organs, arms, legs, and every cell, resulting in the human body and mind becoming "enlightened." The entirety of the ocean flows through us rather than just a stream, and we identify with the ocean, rather than the human form.

However, the concept of a linear path, in which kundalini rises up the body to meet its end goal, is a bit too simplistic. Insofar as the chakra system consists of different levels of consciousness through which the kundalini rises, there also exist initiatory knots, called *granthis* in some yogic systems. Once pierced by kundalini, these knots unravel, allowing a clear passage.

We already have the energetic anatomy to support kundalini streaming through our midline, but like kundalini, this is mostly latent. If the stream is dried up, in order to have ocean water fill it again it may need to be deepened or widened, or to have its structural integrity shored up. Many people who have one explosion out of the top of their head assume that they have had a "kundalini awakening" and that their process is complete, when what they have experienced is a widening of the channel in the midline so that eventually kundalini can flow through.

If we picture the chakra system as initiatory gates through which kundalini will pass, allowing further passage to the higher chakras, we can imagine that kundalini can get fully blocked at any of the gates. It also may have a partial blockage through that gateway. For example, we may develop a substantial flow into the first chakra, with a much smaller flow going into the second. This is because there are still substantial blockages in the first chakra, but no longer enough that kundalini is completely stuck there. In my first book, *The Spiritual Awakening Guide*, I likened this to stones and boulders in a stream. If we have a huge boulder of trauma in our first chakra, it is going to take a lot of time and energy for that stream to do anything but hit that boulder in an effort to eventually wear it down. If it erodes into a large stone rather than a boulder, some of the stream can make its way past.

Even temporary realization of kundalini awakening through the system, feeling that type of flow, can revolutionize and shift our perspective into greater consciousness. But it is not the entirety of the path, and the low level of discourse on kundalini has led people to misunderstand this concept.

If we go back to discussing the chakra system, we do not move through it in a linear fashion, either. Kundalini does not awaken, work its way through everything held in the first chakra, and then move forward to release everything in the second chakra, and so forth.

Working through the Sheaths

Our chakras have layers, commonly referred to as *sheaths*. To return to our metaphor of kundalini energy being like a giant ocean and the possibility of some of that flowing through our midline, it may be a single drop or the entirety of that ocean. It may also divert into a different stream, creating instability, which will be discussed later.

For most of us, we will work our way through one of the sheaths of the chakra first. This means a small stream of energy, even though it feels quite powerful and even volcanic, has made its way from the original ocean and is flowing enough to reach the first or possibly second chakra.

Even if kundalini has awakened, its full potential may not be expressed. This means that a small stream, rather than the full flow of oceanic kundalini, will be rising through our systems. To experience the full ocean of kundalini requires for the three and a half "curls" of kundalini to unravel and straighten. Before this time, we may only be experiencing a fraction of that original ocean, even with the experience of severe symptoms. Due to blockages in our first chakra we can experience even a small stream of kundalini energy emerging as destructive or overwhelming.

In this case we can experience extraordinary heat, itching of the genitals, as well as a high sex drive, to the point of it interfering with our lives. We may end up releasing the energy downwards, through orgasm, instead of purifying and transmuting that sexual essence upwards, leading to transformed consciousness.

Each chakra has several sheaths, and as we work through them more and more of the ocean can emerge and flow through. The first sheath of the first chakra is likely to be about our personal and sexual histories—the sort of abuses and early childhood experiences that are the domain of psychological understanding.

Other sheaths of the first chakra have to do with releasing traumas regarding familial relations, sexual identity, ancestry, past lives, and experiences with birth. The last sheaths are typically more existential, concerning how selfish and narcissistic we are, or the deepest layers of karma, such as the harm that we have enacted against others. Working with the *persecutor* in the last sheaths, we are dealing with the dark and neglected aspects of ourselves that are not socially, personally, or morally correct, as well as our atavistic, animalistic inclinations such as violence and greed.

To return to our stream analogy, that stream can work its way through a sheath or layer of the first chakra and then move on to the second chakra, working on one of its sheaths. Thus we gradually raise our consciousness and take the "elevator" up the midline to have an initial experience of ego death, which is the rising of kundalini energy through the crown.

We may also have a volcanic explosion of kundalini energy through our midline to either prepare the path for kundalini to fully stream through, or to release a sheath, or many sheaths at once. Kundalini is likely then to go back to either a latent state (back to the first chakra) or to more of a stream-like state that is not as intense. Such explosions are rarely necessary, and although they do lead to shifts in consciousness that can be quite dramatic, they can be traumatizing, with a lot of material coming up that needs to be processed and integrated by the system.

The initial stage of kundalini awakening is often referred to as a "purifying fire." This force burns through us, often quite painfully, consuming what prevents us from understanding who we are and our vital connections to the divine, to the earth, and to one another. Past traumas emerge and old emotions surface.

The spiritual awakening process is traumatizing in and of itself, even though it is quite freeing. There is often immense grief, guilt, or realization that our former selves acted in ways that our new selves would never do. It is also quite a shock, on multiple levels, to find ourselves in a space beyond what we once considered to be "truth" or to radically change personal identity and belief systems. It takes a considerable amount of time to reorient the body and mind around the new self, one that no longer holds such heavy beliefs that once made up the core of our identity.

If we understand that this process has many layers, and we imagine a sort of stream that widens and deepens to eventually contain the entirety of the ocean flowing through it, we can move beyond the idea that one tsunami in our system means a highly conscious state. We can then begin to see how kundalini ebbs and flows as it works its way through the chakra system.

The key is to look at how kundalini manifests in the system at the moment. What is its baseline of energy? If there are still blockages in the first chakra, even if the kundalini has flowed through the head momentarily, that means that we are still in the first chakra stage of kundalini awakening. If kundalini has emerged and has a powerful flow into the first chakra, and a small stream going upwards, that means that it has worked through one or two of the sheaths of the first chakra, and is likely working through the first sheath of the second or third chakra.

We can see additional layers of complexity if we look at the larger flows that can either purge the system or ready it for further awakening. If an ocean flows with a tsunami-like force and erupts out of the top of the head but in its baseline state merely trickles through the first chakra, we are likely to bring whatever experiences we have had into the realm of the first chakra and become imbalanced through self-aggrandizement. We may also find that part of the stream has not fully come back to its source. Due to the boulders and eddies of the stream, an eruption of the energy can cause a small stream of kundalini to be stuck in the throat chakra, for instance, while the baseline energy is still in the first chakra. This trapped energy can create a lot of imbalances, physically, emotionally, and spiritually.

It is essential to work through whatever imbalances are held in the area of discomfort due to the kundalini process. We can always be led by our wounds, by what is unhealed within, or by the force within us that desires health, balance, and evolution. To look with clarity at our experiences or find a teacher who can help us to see our blind spots is always a necessity on this path. There is a danger all along the path, especially in heightened states, of feeling superior because we no longer participate in the noise and chaos, the projection and drama that most people fill their days with. It is especially difficult when we begin to feel a fuller flow of kundalini, as people are attracted to this type of energy; there are teachers who have not worked through the final sheath of the first chakra, and so use attention, acclaim, and reverence from others as an excuse to abuse people or to create new karma or imbalances of power.

Untangling the Knots

We have different "knots" in our system that are essentially initiatory. Working through them signifies a huge shift in consciousness.

In Daoist systems, there are three main chakras, called *dan tiens*. These are located in the lower abdomen, the heart, and the third eye. In yogic and Vedanta-based systems, such as Ramana Maharshi's, we discover a series of knots throughout the human form. In many of these systems there was deliberate obscuration of the location of some of these knots. This is understandable, as people would do things like stretch their tongue or even cut a section off in order to make their way to the knot at the roof of the mouth.

During development in utero, the flow of energy through the midline is separated due to the formation of the mouth. This is one of the hardest areas of the physical form to open due to our physical and energetic structure, and people have gone to great lengths to create flows of energy through the midline and into the brain using the tongue as a bridge.

Today people don't often do things like this. But I do find that many people take words as their own without any type of direct experience. While we certainly understand spiritual knowledge through myth and story, what this often leads to in the modern world is people repeating what prior sages and realized individuals have said without deeper understanding. This is not dissimilar to my experience of a semester of French language in high school. If I were to travel to France, I might be able to find my way to the bathroom or the library, but I wouldn't be able to communicate with any sort of depth with the locals.

There are also people who have used spiritual and religious paths to exacerbate states of mental-emotional imbalance. There are many who use the label "kundalini" because they desire a distraction, or something interesting or advanced to happen in their lives. Others can use the label to prevent themselves from looking at prior trauma or mental-emotional imbalances. The result of any type of spiritual awakening should be greater balance, perspective, and ability to meet the world without projections. In such cases, support from an understanding practitioner might be indicated (how to find a healer and what types of modalities are helpful for spiritual awakening are discussed in later chapters).

In discussing the knots, I will go over the ones that have been personally relevant, as well as those I have seen clinically most often.

The first knot is located in the perineum. When kundalini first awakens, it irritates the perineum and gets pushed up by contraction of the pelvic floor. This can cause a vibratory sensation, itching, or pulsing in the perineum alone or of the entire pelvic floor. This knot automatically releases when there is enough force for the "snake" to pierce through and rise into the pelvic bowl. The initiation of this chakra involves moving beyond using our creative or spiritual energy simply for unconscious sex and procreation; we realize that such an energy can be utilized for higher purposes.

The second knot is in the lower abdomen. This knot releases when most of the sheaths of the first and second chakra are worked through, and a stream of energy is clearly felt into the lower abdomen and sacrum. Our small intestine is our *second brain;* it is a place we commonly hold blocked emotions. With this knot, we move from the basic instincts of sex, procreation, and simply taking from the world into healing aspects of trauma and issues of personal identity.

Before we work our way through this knot, we believe that we are isolated, that we can only count on ourselves to provide nurturing, and we spend a lot of time and energy on the content and creations of our mind. The trauma we have experienced has created a complex series of projections onto the world and the people in it, and it has drastically altered our belief systems. In this state, we continually perpetuate separation, as well as the loops, or repeated behaviors, that have arisen due to trauma.

If our consciousness is located in the first, second and third chakras, our spiritual path is likely to be entirely self-serving. Here we engage with our prior traumas and mental projections, as well as digestive processes and our physical form. This is actually necessary, as the first aspect of any spiritual path should be about personal healing. But this is not the entirety of the spiritual path. As we work through this spiritual knot we realize that there are other sources of nurturing—the earth, other people, the divine.

We also move away from being so identified with the human form and we no longer see it as a means to an end. This is a perspective shift, in which we release the chaos that we have created out of trauma, boredom, and self-obsession.

When we experience trauma, we fracture. The part of ourselves that is traumatized and overwhelmed becomes frozen, a stagnant part of our consciousness. We are populated with frozen aspects of consciousness—an army of unhealed six-year-olds, teenagers, twenty- and thirty-somethings, infants. It is impossible for us to attend to anything else other than our own healing when we have so many frozen aspects of consciousness. They create significant weight and dysfunction. We spend much of our daily lives recreating our trauma in loops (repeated behaviors originating from a traumatic experience) so it can find closure. These frozen aspects of ourselves wish to be seen and heard, to be recognized as a part of the whole again.

They wish to experience *completion of the biological process*, which means closure; such closure is found by allowing expression of emotions that were too overwhelming at the time of the trauma, as well as fulfilling whatever needs that traumatized self may have so it can become unfrozen. It is by healing these frozen aspects of consciousness that we can come into our present-day consciousness, that we can move beyond our wounding and separation and into self-realization, enlightenment, and greater flow. My book *The Body Deva* is designed for people going through spiritual awakenings to help them look towards their bodies to see what traumas are creating a lack of flow and present-day consciousness in their systems.

In addition to our personal traumas, we also have ancestral and past life traumas that are healed by kundalini rising through the first and second chakras. As kundalini works its way through several sheaths, we can recognize our past lives and heal our ancestral wounding. We begin to recognize that we can be nurtured by more than just ourselves.

In this knot, we may experience a momentary ego death, or an explosion of kundalini energy above the head. We see that we are more than just our physical bodies, and a channel opens through which we recognize connection to and nurturing from the divine (or top-down energies).

In my book *The Spiritual Awakening Guide*, I talk about different types of awakenings, including Top-Down Awakenings. They are the most common type of awakening in our culture, and they occur through spiritual pursuits that are ungrounded or simply too intense. We do not like attending to the physical form in a gradual or disciplined way to experience spiritual energies. A top-down awakening is quite different; the third eye and crown chakras are most often activated by differentiated energy or qi, instead of kundalini or the downward flow of grace and connection to spirit and the divine. When this happens without grounding and preparation of the system, and without healing trauma in the first and second chakras, we can become imbalanced. Without the perspective that we should stabilize, ground, and attend to the darker aspects of life, we may lose our tether to reality, or experience headaches or mania due to influxes of psychic energy that has nowhere to flow. Because the throat chakra can open only through a healing of the lower chakras, what happens when the upper psychic centers open is that there is a great deal of differentiated or spiritual energy around the head, with little energy, differentiated or not, in the rest of the body.

The next knot is right above the center of the diaphragm. When opening, it goes through periods of painful contraction, pulsation, as well as body or breath "locks." These are automatic and quite painful experiences of all the breath being exhaled from the body while the solar plexus contracts against the spine. These contractions, involving the spontaneous sucking in of air until the spine flattens, produce large flows of energy throughout the body. This is similar to the contraction and pulsation of the perineum at the activation of kundalini, with the effect of energy being cycled from the solar plexus area into the heart.

With this knot, we realize that others have the same consciousness as ourselves. However, this realization is nuanced. We are all awakened; we just have a lot of junk in the way of that realization and some have less junk than others. This is the first awakening of true compassion, and with the release of this knot we can use the outer world and the people in it to see what still lies unresolved within. The need for spiritual competition and egoic superiority complexes drops away, relationships and interpersonal relationships deepen, and we meet the world and the people in it as they are, not as we would like them to be.

While there is still personal trauma (and the uncovering of last sheaths of the first three chakras) to attend to, we have enough perspective beyond our egoic selves to begin to see and work on the "grids": the collective energies, history, mythology, and larger constructs that create and inform us.

When we begin to move away from our self-obsession, we see that our history, society, culture, world, and cosmic forces have created us. We are no longer enmeshed with these energies and witness them from a place of differentiation. This is popularly known as a deconditioning process, which is quite apt. The initial realization of outlying grids occurs when kundalini energy emerges in the solar plexus area, and it is fully realized in the third eye and by kundalini energy rising into the brain.

When the knot in the third eye is opened, psychic abilities flourish, as do *siddhis*, or powers associated with supernatural elements or capacities to move beyond or master the physical form. There occurs a realization of all timelines, a direct revelation of multiple dimensions, the ability to move beyond humanity and see oneself as part of a web, instead of its center. Consciousness occurs as a direct knowing.

In some traditions, there is also a series of knots that go from the third eye up into the crown that need to be unraveled. They hold us back from undifferentiated consciousness, from Shakti meeting Shiva, from the feminine and masculine duality intertwining and becoming one.

While it is entirely expected and natural to have many ego deaths—bursts or flows above the crown that offer this perspective—when the stream of kundalini flows permanently in some small or large way through the entire midline and up through the head, we recognize and reconcile paradox.

The combination of spiritual energies merging above the head with individual consciousness fully meeting cosmic consciousness, takes us beyond the mind and its dominance. As we work through the forehead knot we find ourselves experiencing paradoxical states. Through the descent of energy into the heart knots, we are simultaneously very human and imperfect, attending to our daily lives, as well as an aspect of cosmic consciousness. We are both a single drop in the ocean that is cosmic consciousness and the entirety of the flow.

The last knot is that of the spiritual heart. There are many knots around the heart and the spiritual heart (the area that surrounds the heart, basically). As we work through these knots we become more and more compassionate to the world around us. With the return of the individual identity, as the flow of grace descends and ascends simultaneously, there is an experience of being a cosmic "I." The huge creative force and potency that is cosmic energy flows through the system; we go from feeling as if we are on an individual path and taking from the world to considering how we can be of benefit to the world.

In this state kundalini is no longer a goddess, feminine, or even kundalini. It is cosmic flow, and recognition of the cosmic "I"—we see how the elements that created us allow us to be of unique benefit to the world. We are informed by "all that is" through our individualized, human vessel. As the energy descends we find ourselves grounded and deeply immersed in the world again. We appreciate the significance of our human forms and their ability to connect on many levels. We traverse the spiritual path for benefit of the world, not for the self.

Additional knots include a knot at the back of the neck that is associated with the brain stem. It is here that a great deal of our self-hatred lies; releasing this knot involves accepting all aspects of self on all levels. It doesn't mean changing any emotions or experience, but a deep acceptance of them. This is an incredibly difficult knot for people to work through. Accounts of St. Teresa of Avila, Buddha, and other spiritual figures fighting a final battle—with their minds, with outer demons or inner parasites—might refer to working through this knot. Releasing this knot allows for kundalini to flow through and into the brain, where light expands. While some people going through spiritual awakenings focus on the pineal gland, the third ventricle, or activation of the *bindu* point, kundalini eventually flows through the entirety of the brain.

There is also a knot in the roof of the mouth, as previously mentioned. Located above the vomer bone (the indent near the top of the mouth) it allows for kundalini to flow through the throat into the internal structures of the brain. In CranioSacral therapy, the throat is referred to as the *avenue of expression*, and in Chinese medicine there is a channel that originates in the heart and flows through the tongue, allowing someone to express their soul authentically and clearly to the world. We often have a lot of fear and trauma about doing this, and it can be a hard pathway to open. There are methods in qi gong and yoga to press the tip of the tongue against the roof of the mouth to create a bridge between the throat and the brain so that kundalini can flow through that bridge.

We might experience a feeling of sinus release, or a dripping of "nectar" or cerebrospinal fluid from the tongue spontaneously pressing the roof of the mouth or thrusting in a variety of ways. The tongue thrusting, spontaneous vocalization, and contracture of the throat to achieve a permanent state of flow are quite odd, as are spontaneous vocalizations and the emergence of divinely inspired creative pursuits. Once this knot is opened the authentic cosmic "I" that has been awakened in the spiritual heart has a clear pathway to bring itself into the world.

As you can see, kundalini awakening is an intensive and often difficult process, with many layers and stages. It is by educating ourselves, by being willing to see with clarity where we are in the process, that we can move beyond simple or intellectualized concepts and into direct experience, revelation, and liberation.

5

Why and How
Kundalini Awakens

While there have been attempts to describe kundalini as a neurological process, specifically one having to do with the vagus nerve, this is not an either/or proposition. Rather, it is a physiological and spiritual process simultaneously, as we exist on a continuum, our physical aspects simply being the most dense.

The kundalini awakening process is one of neurological rewiring that involves deep shifts in the neuro-endocrine system. This rewiring occurs so that the intensifying spiritual power can flow through the system.

Our spiritual nervous system (which includes the chakra system and physical nervous system) is our first interface with any type of spiritual energy. It provides an avenue for differentiated energy, filters it, and allows kundalini to rise through it. If there is an overload of this system (due to physical injury, trauma and emotional dysregulation, sensitivity or interface with initiatory experiences that create large shifts in consciousness, or continual immersion without a filter) there is disruption to all aspects of the continuum that is the nervous system—spiritual, energetic, emotional, and physical.

Kundalini awakening is highly disruptive to the digestive system, as well as to the neurological and endocrine systems. There is some discussion amongst contemporary scientists about how our DNA can be altered by traumatic experiences. In addition, studies on the brains of long-term meditators point to the impact of spiritual experiences on the physical form. However, we are unlikely to truly understand consciousness and the impact of spiritual activity until mind, body, and spirit are seen as a continuum, not as separate things. Our current materialist paradigms can measure or sense only a small fraction of the spiritual layers of reality.

It can be difficult at first to see the difference between a nervous system that is hyperreactive or dysfunctional due to trauma and one going through a rewiring or purification process as a result of kundalini awakening. This can be exacerbated by people who have decided that they are experiencing a kundalini awakening because they have physical damage to the nervous system or may be experiencing mental-emotional imbalances and wish to grasp onto the "kundalini" label so as to not need to fully contend with the reality of their situation.

It is necessary to look at the overall trajectory of the spiritual path, rather than merely symptoms. The expansion of consciousness and a movement away from self-obsession are what result from the initial phase; everything else is a byproduct. If there is no expansion of consciousness occurring, we are either stuck in initial stages of the kundalini awakening process or not experiencing kundalini awakening. If someone has awakened kundalini through emotional or physical trauma, which is a common antecedent for awakening (thus confusing things even further), the first phase of the kundalini awakening process should focus on nervous system repair, re-regulation, and healing of trauma.

The first phase of kundalini awakening is a purifying process in which the personal history, wounds, and emotional issues emerge. Sometimes we blame meditation, yoga or kundalini itself for being the cause of emotional imbalances. What happens through any meditative or kundalini awakening process is the emergence of trauma held in the subconscious. Prior to the process we were reacting to it, living it out in repetitive loops; the flow of kundalini simply unearths these held energies and static forms of consciousness and brings them into conscious awareness. We were already experiencing the impact of the held trauma, but it had not yet come into conscious awareness.

People often assume that meditation and spiritual activities will automatically make them feel better. Many of us crave a healthy form of being. With the popularity of things like mindfulness, we sometimes come in with the belief that the result should be pleasant, or a kind of numbness.

The purpose of meditation can be many things. Self-realization is high on that list, as are liberation and enlightenment. One prominent objective would be to release whatever arises in the mind. Our minds are filled with noise created by what lies unhealed within us; by allowing these noises to be heard, we can move beyond them and then find ourselves in the present moment. If we heal the past, we no longer project into the future, and find ourselves with a clear, bright mind that is interested and immersed in the present moment.

Another purpose would be mental training. If we understand our minds and how they work, we can understand our reasons for being the way we are. We can see our loops (repeated behaviors arising from trauma) clearly, and move beyond them. We can experience our minds working for us or with us, instead of against us.

By understanding how we fit into social and cultural paradigms, we can decondition the mind and reckon with the atavistic aspects of self. The objective is not to never have a thought again, but to be fully conscious and to think dynamically, creatively, and fruitfully, without the noise of trauma or social conditioning.

In the West, we tend to segment spiritual knowledge. A proper education in meditation would include both focusing (contraction) as well as depth or expansion. Present moment awareness, mantras, and other methods bring us into clarity and offer us the ability to see sharply. Self-inquiry, such as *The Body Deva* method, allow us to see our motivations for being. Doing present moment awareness methods without self-inquiry would be like sitting at a lake in which we just see the surface twinkling. We may be in the present moment, we may be focused, but we are not healing or resolving much within.

Similarly, if we are just doing self-inquiry, we may know our motivations for being, but we may not have the focus and presence to stabilize what is being unearthed within us. This would be like continually dredging up sludge from the bottom of that lake without seeing its beauty, or not realizing that the spiritual path can be more than a Sisyphean effort with little reward.

In meditation we turn inward and create a space in which what has been held within, which is often traumatized, fearful, angry, or grieving, can rise into consciousness. This can involve some degree of pain, or at the very least some unpleasant emotions.

It is only by passing through these emotions that the mind starts to quiet. Meditation is mind training. Just as we learn to take care of our physical forms—through exercise, nutrition, and so on—our mind requires education as well, specifically the skills and tools that meditation can uniquely offer. Daily meditation over a lengthy period of time is really the only way to awaken beyond the first knot.

I do realize that many people wish to be advanced or far along their path with little or no effort, or wish to simply feel better, or to not feel anything at all, as a result of their efforts. Our society encourages this, due to our incredibly imbalanced view of the purpose and expression of the emotions. We may see our emotions as "bad," and believe that if we just "transcend" them we will never feel pain, anger, or grief. There are entire communities where people wear masks, pretending that they do not feel anything but "love" and "light." In this illusion, love is seen as the only valid emotion, and all other emotions and experiences are something to disregard, villainize, or transmute into love, often through rather harsh means.

All of our emotions are vital messengers. It is by being loving towards all aspects of ourselves that we can awaken beyond these illusions and masks. For instance, rather than transmute anger into love, we see it as a sacred gift with a purpose. The spiritual awakening process allows us to feel more dynamically our full range of emotions. We can actually see others, care for them, and experience our emotions dynamically, without stopping, harassing, or forcing them to be something that they are not.

The churning in the initial stages of a kundalini awakening of what has been held within the channels and chakras is often very hard on us, especially if we were not mentally-emotionally balanced prior to our spiritual experiences. This is why attending to trauma and personal healing is suggested before doing anything in regards to the kundalini awakening itself.

We must be stable mentally, emotionally, and physically for kundalini to rise correctly. Otherwise we can get lost in seeing our experiences through the lens of trauma. We can get stuck in the first chakra needs of being seen as superior, worthy, or special. Any spiritual experiences can become fuel for creating further imbalance, rather than a movement towards health.

There is a very real question of how many in our world have a truly functioning and healthy nervous system. We are a culture that very much is centered around *doing*. We hold ourselves to psychological ideals regarding normalcy and health, yet we live in a world thick with trauma where few of us function in our adult capacity. Rare is the nervous system that can appropriately shift from a fight or flight state to a rest and digest state, switching from the sympathetic system to the parasympathetic in a healthy manner.

Another profound shift that occurs as a result of the kundalini awakening process is a complete rerouting of the digestive fire. There can be lengthy periods of dysfunction and ill health due to this rerouting.

If kundalini is most active in our first and second chakras, we will have dysfunction in those areas. If this is a small stream, this discomfort may be minimal. If this is the whole force of the ocean slamming against a wall in the first chakra, there may be issues with the genitals, gynecological problems possibly including endometriosis and pain and emotionality prior to, during, and after the menstrual cycle, and lower digestive tract issues.

If we are experiencing a kundalini awakening we will feel where kundalini is working, sometimes as dysfunction or pain for a period of time and then a resolution of symptoms. The kundalini energy then moves on to the next "boulder" or next area of the body to work on. This can be quite a sudden shift, with a felt sensation that kundalini energy is completing work in a specific portion of the body and moving on to the next one. Spiritual illness and physical illness often appear very differently; spiritual illness tends to arise suddenly, painfully, and mysteriously, and disappear with that same nature.

While sometimes we can experience small streams or creeping sensations of heat-based energy, this can also be quite dramatic. For example, we can experience a shift from immense pain in the hip with sensations of volcanic heat and rising of trauma and held emotions from that area, to a sensation of kundalini working in the diaphragm with that same intensity, with prior hip pain dissolving.

Sometimes we assume that kundalini awakening means that we will have perfect health. While this process can resolve old symptoms, including physical ones, it is helpful to keep in mind that quite realized people in history, such as Ramana Maharshi and Krishnamurti, died of cancer.

What does happen is that symptoms change. Diagnoses can also change, particularly of functional disorders such as chronic fatigue, some of the autoimmune diseases, and other endocrine and nervous system issues. It is typical for people experiencing kundalini to have to deal with often strange health issues; we then need to discern whether the pain or symptoms will resolve when kundalini has moved on from working in a particular area or if we should explore allopathic treatment.

How Kundalini Arises

Kundalini arises through the cerebrospinal matrix; our cerebrospinal fluid creates a pathway that goes through the spinal canal and bathes the brain. In many ways, CranioSacral therapy is the perfect modality for working with kundalini awakenings, as here the focus is on the cerebrospinal fluid, as well as the linings and osseous structures of the skull and spinal canal.

The Upledger form of CranioSacral therapy also works intraorally, which is incredibly helpful for those who have blockages in the throat or who are at the point where kundalini is attempting to rise through the tongue into the brain.

The stream of kundalini goes through the spinal canal to pass through the ventricular system of the brain, particularly the third ventricle. This ventricle lights up when kundalini rises through the tongue and into the middle of the brain, going through the knot that is located near the vomer. This results in an opening of that knot and cerebrospinal fluid dripping down into the digestive system, resolving or lessening the significant digestive distress that often occurs in kundalini awakenings.

There is a focus on the pineal gland in popular culture with regard to awakenings. It is difficult to ascribe authenticity to the reports of experiences from use of DMT and other psychedelics, because prior knowledge and interest in popular culture is a lens that can heavily filter the user's experience. Kundalini rising into the brain seems to eventually be a brain-wide activity, including many structures, particularly those in the midbrain. As most people are unable to achieve kundalini rising into the brain on a permanent basis (rather than a temporary explosion or occasional stream) receiving enough reliable reports to note overall tendencies is difficult if not impossible.

The permanent flow of kundalini into the brain would seemingly give us complete power over our autonomic nervous system. This includes the ability to stop and start our pulse at will, huge creative flows, and genius level aptitude at our unique potential. Yogis who have reached this state can consciously decide when their time of death will be; they can project their energy out of the *bindu* point at the time of their chosen release of the physical form. Even experiencing a temporary flow into the brain can allow for huge creative potential, such as the ability to write a book within a week.

Mania can also allow for bursts of creative energy; often the difference has to do with whether the work is focused on the self or on something useful for others. If there is a downward flow of spiritual energy without a flow of spiritual energy from the root chakra coming up, we can experience huge creative flows but the result is through the lens of trauma, mental-emotional imbalance, and self-obsession. This is akin to the person declaring that they are the Messiah and that their five thousand-page text is their decree that everyone in the world should follow.

Others have postulated that kundalini awakenings have to do with blood, DNA, and lymphatic fluid in the body. This idea was especially espoused by Gopi Krishna, who believed that there was a genetic component to kundalini awakening; it was something that was either passed down the familial systems or through DNA and it expressed itself through the blood.

Generally I have found that kundalini does express itself through the fluid systems of the body. Women who have experienced severe menstrual cramps and other difficulties have found that rerouting the energy properly and resolving held trauma in the sacral area caused many of their symptoms to decrease or disappear. Others found that more physical aspects of their hormonal or menstrual cycles simply functioned better than they had before.

Some occult traditions point to our spiritual power being held in the blood. Sacrifice of animals as well as humans in certain societies demonstrates how the spilling of blood, and its link and usage to spiritual or magical power, has been known by many disparate cultures. Even today in some occult or esoteric circles there is consideration of the power of blood, where it is viewed as a powerful and dangerous fuel for spiritual workings.

The Wise Wound by Penelope Shuttle and Peter Redgrave is a poetic (and rather out of date scientifically) book that discusses the inherent power of women and the menstrual cycle—the feminine creative capacity that we all emerge from—in the context of a patriarchal society that wishes to diminish this power. We can look towards spiritual traditions that understand that blood contains the essence of our power, and understand how kundalini (spiritual power) can easily create dysfunction and dysregulation within blood and lymphatic systems in its initial attempts to rise and flow.

Why Kundalini Arises

I am continually asked why kundalini emerges. How can someone who has done yoga for forty years never experience an awakening, while someone else can have a spontaneous awakening and even sudden self-realization?

The simple answer seems to be prior life preparations. One of my first spiritual teachers told this joke: *If you want to awaken, start meditating now and in three lifetimes of daily cultivation you will awaken.* This is something that most people do not wish to hear. The spiritual path takes effort; even if you pursue it whole-heartedly or go live as an ascetic for fifty years, you may not reach an enlightened state. The good news is that many of us have made substantial efforts in previous lives, though we may not be aware of them consciously.

But if we consider that a yogi who has maintained a strict practice of disciplined devotion through an authentic lineage of gurus and within a social construct that still considers the spiritual as part of daily, lived reality may not have reached enlightenment through his *tapasya* of holding one arm upward consistently for forty years, our modern Western illusions become readily apparent.

Even with past life efforts, higher consciousness states cannot be achieved or maintained without dedicated effort. It is not difficult to find peak experiences through psychedelics, sensory deprivation, or military-like meditation retreats. That is not to say that these are not useful experiences. They can tell the body that such states are possible by recognizing, even for a moment, what is obscuring the realized state; from that perspective, however momentary it is, we realize that we do not need to hang on to our wounding. We may also perceive the larger forces governing our reality and in some small way decondition ourselves from those forces.

But there is a difference between a temporary experience and a permanent state. The spiritual path will naturally weed out those who prefer illusion to the dedication and effort required to truly become more conscious. We live in a world where there is such disregard for the spiritual that it has created teachers who haven't been students, and what is illusory is so tempting because it isn't real. Such dreams and fantastical illusions will always be superior to any type of reality, and they perpetuate the type of spiritual emptiness that is so pervasive in our world instead of healing it.

There is much to be said for preparing the system for kundalini to awaken. Many schools of yoga as well as meditative and spiritual paths balance and ready the system for kundalini to awaken. Through readying of the appropriate physical and psychic structures within the body for kundalini to awaken, the experience of kundalini arising can be less difficult.

It would be wonderful to understand why kundalini emerges in every system, particularly those of us who have not developed the appropriate energetic container beforehand (a lengthy period in a pre-kundalini state, or awakening of differentiated qi energies flowing through the meridians of the body) or who are not emotionally or physically prepared for such an opening. What I have found is that spirit sometimes defies expectation.

Many of us who experience kundalini awakenings do so because of a yearning to experience divinity. A deep hunger for the divine, even on a subconscious level, seems to propel many of us. Those who look for more existential qualities, such as truth, connection, knowledge, or who strive to understand the spiritual experiences they've already had, do at the very least tend to move away from self-obsession.

There are also people who for whatever reason are awake from an early age and their spiritual experiences were nurtured rather than pathologized. At the age of six most of us go to school and begin a long process of socialization outside of our families, in which many expectations of normalcy are placed on us. Even those of us who are awake or have anything approaching high perception feel the need to wear a mask, or to deny aspects of ourselves, to fit into our daily environments.

Other Models of Kundalini

There have been other routes suggested for kundalini awakening through the system. When the word *kundalini* came into greater awareness in the West, there were models, most significantly the one by Itzhak Bentov in his work *Stalking the Wild Pendulum*, that found that modern Western people first felt the energy in their feet, where it would rise up the body through the back of the body and then come down the front, ending in the abdomen. He wondered why people had such different, or more significant experiences of kundalini awakening outside of modern Western culture.

Such a model often points to the preparatory phase, or pre-kundalini, where differentiated energy (qi) begins to open the meridians. This type of awakening is much more common than kundalini awakenings.

Pre-kundalini states do need quite a bit of guidance and assistance; such a process is often painful and leads to shifts in identity and the release of held trauma. If it does not involve the midline, the drastic evolution of consciousness that is the marker of kundalini awakening does not occur. Sushumna (the central channel) is the controller of all of the other channels of the body, and it is by kundalini arising through it that our consciousness truly unfolds.

Various teachers claim that kundalini can be awakened through the knot located under the belly button. I have never found much evidence for this. Others talk about an outer force, such as a lightning bolt (metaphorically or literally), a dynamic experience of self-realization that comes in through the crown with such force that kundalini is sparked. Some equate this to the Holy Spirit. This is the masculine pole moving towards the feminine, and with enough authenticity in a primed system we can experience the merging of the feminine and masculine, leading to a realized state.

However, most people experiencing top-down energies are not sparking kundalini. Instead they may be opening the psychic centers of the head with differentiated energy that has nowhere to go, leading to imbalance. Spiritual energy that flows through the top down is not integrated into daily reality and through all layers of our being (mind, body, spirit). For balance to occur we must open from the root chakra upwards; otherwise we are looking at reality through a limited lens.

It can be tempting to focus on the symptoms of awakening, especially the loud ones—doing spontaneous backbends or having enormous shaking go through your system is quite fascinating for good reason. However, the best way to assess kundalini awakening is through the expansion of consciousness over time, the lessening of trauma and emotional patterns of wounding, and the development of greater stability.

It should also be pointed out that we can have a transcendental moment that immensely shifts our world view. This can occur in nature, through spiritual or magical ritual, or with plant medicines. In a prepared and ready soul, this can only assist evolution and the awakening process. If we have limited consciousness, we will often grasp onto such experiences, creating feelings of superiority or being special with no greater consciousness being attained.

On Surrender

Surrendering on deeper and deeper levels is in many ways the only advice needed in any spiritual process.

The advice to surrender does not mean that we do nothing. It has been taken this way in the modern world due to ignorance. We can only surrender what is held within us—what is obscuring our awakened state— by active participation in our own process. Otherwise what can emerge are the horror stories we hear, typically from individuals without a proper framework or guidance. Kundalini is never really the problem; it is what has been conditioned in our minds that creates all of the ruckus.

Our resistance is what is unhealed within us, it is our mind, our ego; it has a vested interest in our reality remaining as it is and will fight for its needs to be met. We are also incredibly traumatized in the modern world because we are so disconnected. Our natural connections and cycling of energy with the natural world, with other people, with ourselves, and with divinity have been disrupted. In such a disconnected state, we have nothing to surrender to. We believe that there is nothing that will nurture us, including ourselves. It is only by actively participating in our own process—by training our mind, by being willing to see where we are on our spiritual path with clarity, and by healing trauma—that it becomes possible for us to step out of our way.

As we step more and more into our present-day consciousness, and as what has been frozen inside of us comes into an adult capacity and the present moment, we have the capacity to move towards health. It is by engaging with the health of our systems, by healing trauma, that we can begin to reconnect again. By doing so we are no longer drowning in our lives. Not only are we willing and eager to participate in the evolution of our own consciousness, but we can surrender. We do so without fear, understanding that such a surrender can only benefit us.

Illusion and Kundalini

It is very true that those who have devoted themselves to a spiritual path or who have authentically experienced a kundalini awakening cannot fully describe just how difficult such a path is. Kundalini awakenings require a great deal of sacrifice. In return we receive greater stillness and perspective; the weight of past trauma diminishes.

At every stage of the path we are met by the illusion that we are much further along than we are. So many confuse the initial spark of anything spiritual for enlightenment, and many others confuse illusions created from a separated self that craves spirit, magic, and connection to something greater than itself.

We are so devoid of magic, of spirit, in our world that even a drop of it is taken on by the thirsty soul. We find what we are ready for. We find what we are looking for. If you continually question what you are looking for, and understand that the ego creates fear and mythic illusions, we can see this ego trick each time for what it is. Thinking we are further on the path than we are is a form of resistance to keep us where we are. Daily self-inquiry, such as working with *The Body Deva*, can allow us to see what is still unresolved within us.

In authentic awakenings of any type we can recognize the shift in perspective, the realization that we are simply a drop in the ocean. When the illusion of the ego is seen through, it is impossible for us to feel in control or superior to anything. We begin to realize how little we know.

We can also look for a release of former patterns, greater connection to the self, the world, and the people in it, and a general sense of ease, as well as stillness. The spiritual process should make us eventually more stable, more functional, and better able to interact with anyone we choose. It is not a process of disconnection, of isolating in a bubble, or of removing anything that is irritating from our life. Many spiritual teachers have obnoxious or irritating students who they specifically want in their spiritual communities because it allows the other students to see what they still need to resolve within. This cannot happen if the student puts themselves in a bubble that does not contain any difficult or irritating elements.

6

Pre-kundalini and Neuro-kundalini

There is a rather trite metaphor about the spiritual path being like climbing a mountain; there are many paths up the mountain and many different ways of walking the spiritual path. This is quite apt, and it is reasonable to suggest that any spiritual path involves kundalini awakening in some regard. We could also make the argument that any activity, particle, cell, artistic endeavor, or body function is a result of kundalini. However, what most people confuse for kundalini awakening are pre-kundalini states, or nervous system dysregulation due to trauma or traumatic injury (neuro-kundalini).

To continue the metaphor, about halfway up said mountain all of us, no matter the path, will begin to feel the expression and awakening of kundalini. However, some of us start our spiritual paths quite suddenly, without any type of spiritual discipline or understanding, and that path is quite a bit rockier. To be able to handle it properly, we need to play a bit of catch-up to that halfway point as kundalini energy has already expressed in our system.

Typically the first stage of any spiritual path focuses on self-healing and trauma care because it is necessary to heal in order to be willing to nurture ourselves. If we are traumatized, we are resistant and unable to take care of our mind, body, and spirit; that resistance lessens the more we heal.

Going through a kundalini awakening without any prior preparation leaves us far less able to handle a volcanic explosion through our system than someone who has been gradually exploring a disciplined spiritual, bodywork, or meditative path and finds themselves mid-mountain after twenty years. Learning cultivation and establishing an appropriate physical and energetic container for kundalini to awaken within the body while simultaneously going through a kundalini awakening can be quite difficult to accomplish.

If we are able to become aware of past lives we can bring the past cultivation and spiritual knowledge gathered in them into conscious awareness. Ironically, recalling past lives to the extent that their benefits come through, rather than the lingering traumas, seems to primarily happen when kundalini has reached the third eye area, long past the time when we needed such knowledge. However, looking towards past efforts at cultivation in previous lifetimes can allow us to continue on an already established path that was interrupted by physical death.

The path of awakening looks different for each of us, although there are markers we can all recognize along the path. The aspect of ourselves that has been neglected is the one that is the most likely to have difficulties and that is the signpost for where we need to focus our attention. If we have an imbalanced physical form while awakening, our primary difficulties will manifest in the physical. If we lack emotional intelligence, this imbalance will be dominant on the spiritual path. Or we may get fascinated and entrenched in simply having a spiritual experience. We may not be able to reconcile having a spiritual experience in the modern world; there is a battle between the parts of ourselves that know that something extraordinary is happening in our lives, and the parts who are hanging on to wanting a simple, normal existence.

Pre-kundalini states involve an activation of qi as it cycles through the channels (meridians) of the body. This can occur through pursuits like meditation, bodywork, energy work, and yoga. Because this creates symptoms like body twitches or even spontaneous body movements, it is easy to confuse the release of trauma-based energy or held emotions through the nervous system, or the opening and cycling of the channels, for kundalini awakening. This is an activation of the more surface-level, differentiated energy within our systems. This type of awakening can give way eventually to kundalini experiences; during pre-kundalini the channels open and churn, beginning to release and rebalance the channels in the body as a whole. That way the system is prepared for kundalini awakening.

The opening of the acupuncture channels and movement of energy through them is an important initial stage of awakening. Buzzing, twitching, and feelings of electrical activity that can be quite painful mean that the meridians are opening up, widening for kundalini energy to eventually flow through. In this stage we may have spiritual experiences, and momentary spiritual connections and realizations, that point to our body going through a cultivation process.

In Chinese medicine, channels are referred to as "regular" and "extraordinary." Someone experiencing neuro-kundalini or pre-kundalini is likely to experience energy flowing through the primary or regular meridians of the body, such as twitching or heat in the hands, legs, and feet. We have a few different extraordinary meridians, but the ones we are most concerned with in kundalini awakenings are the *du* and *ren*, which circle from the genitals up the back on the midline, and then come back down to the genital area through the front.

Kundalini awakening happens through spiritual energy flowing up the midline, and it is only when kundalini pierces through the chakras, organs, and energetic structures in the midline, that the nervous system can be re-wired and consciousness can truly unfold. While there can be a mild heat, emotional release, twitches and even body movements with pre- and neuro-kundalini, we do not experience the large changes in consciousness that occur with kundalini flowing up through the midline. While certainly there is qi circulation through all of our meridians, including our extraordinary ones, there is a degree of flow and heat as well as a centering of activity in the midline that will not be had by those experiencing pre-kundalini states.

One of the difficulties in describing such a differentiation is that if we have not directly experienced kundalini awakening, we can easily confuse the sensations of qi moving through the body, or of nervous system activation, for kundalini awakenings.

Discerning someone who is mentally-emotionally imbalanced or has nervous system dysregulation from kundalini awakening is further complicated by the fact that many of us awaken through physical or mental-emotional trauma. Trauma has a way of cracking us open psychically; we can become hypersensitive and reactive to the world, with a dysregulated nervous system that now feels as if everyone and everything is a threat to its very survival. Such mechanisms are often forged in early childhood, especialy if abuse by a parent or caregiver is prevalent.

Gabor Mate talks a great deal about the link between trauma and autoimmune states. If we experience trauma in early childhood it sets us up to battle ourselves, as well as to battle the outer world. We may create mythologies that great spiritual forces, including kundalini, are engaging us in a battle. It is only by understanding this inner battle and recognizing where it stems from that we diminish the need for it.

In examining psychosis and the spiritual awakening process, John Weir Perry found that there was frequently a schism between the archetypal or mythic self and the inner reality of such individuals. They were creating myths regarding themselves and the outer world; they view themselves as prophets, enlightened, or great seers in diametrical opposition to their inner reality of feeling small, traumatized, and worthless.

Such individuals find themselves at the center of a process of mythological proportions in which they need to usher in a new world, or they are at the center of battle of good versus evil, or all the evil in the Universe is after them personally. These individuals may be experiencing some sort of spiritual awakening process authentically, such as neuro-kundalini, kundalini emerging and trapped in the first chakra, or kundalini rising up the *pingala* channel (discussed later). But without the proper grounding in collective reality, their insights are likely to be self-serving, and their progress on the spiritual path will be minimal.

Our mythologies and the mythological layers of existence must be anchored into our daily reality. Myth connects us to greater spiritual reality and to the archetypal levels of existence. We can relate to the archetypal figure of Atlas who holds the weight of the world on his shoulders because we also feel this weight. Through myth and archetype we can move beyond the isolation that trauma and struggle create and into seeing the shared human experience.

We can also use myth to point to the ineffable experiences that we have when we are in communion with the spiritual. In this way myth, archetype, and symbol create a bridge between our daily reality and spiritual reality. If our myths are a result of trauma or mental-emotional projections, they serve to separate us further from reality and from authentic communion with the spiritual layers of reality. If our mythologies and archetypes are a functional bridge, they serve to connect us to one another, as well as to the spiritual realms.

There are many ways that we can awaken: for instance, near-death or death experiences, long-term meditation, sexual practices that cultivate energy, plant medicines and hallucinogens, flotation tanks, long-term holistic or therapeutic care, past life or ancestral predisposition, trauma, and yearning to find something greater than the self. In authentic spiritual awakening processes, we move beyond seeing ourselves as the center of the Universe. This does not mean the end of any or all difficulties, or perfect health. But there is a specific kind of shift in perspective, as well as emotional and spiritual shifts, that make us more functional. We become better able to meet the world and the people in it in an adult capacity. In such states, we see ourselves as part of a web, rather than its center.

In states such as psychosis or other unhealed or rigid mental states there is a distinct lack of nuance; things are either black and white, evil or good. We are the eternal victim with a casting of outer villains.

The spiritual path allows us to see and experience nuance rather than polarities. However, a path towards greater wholeness, with its experience of nuance, can only be seen over lengthy periods of time, and it is good to be cautious about labeling anything outside of cultural norms as psychosis or mental illness.

For someone with a dysregulated or non-functional nervous system, the impact of qi moving through the system, with the subsequent release of emotions and held trauma, can be quite traumatic. When an emotionally out of balance or highly traumatized individual experiences awakening when they were already overwhelmed by the contents of their psyche, the experience of kundalini awakening can easily create more trauma, further struggle to manage daily existence, or result in the creation of ungrounded mythic realities to separate the individual further from their lives.

Those who experience physical trauma, as well as states of dysautonomia, may be mistaking nervous system difficulties for kundalini awakening. Alternatively, as a result of a near-death experience, physical trauma or brain injury, we may begin to awaken.

For someone who has experienced trauma due to physical injury, attempting to heal from the ensuing trauma and shock, and grappling with the physical reality of the situation is already difficult. Having either qi awakening, pre-kundalini or kundalini awakening occurring simultaneously or as a result of the experience can create further chaos and confusion for a system that is attempting to figure out the best avenue to heal itself.

In cases of traumatic brain injury or awakening due to trauma it is typical to experience neuro-kundalini symptoms, specifically in the areas of the body that were damaged due to the trauma. While this can lead to kundalini awakening and the expansion of consciousness, what most often happens is that any spiritual energy that has been stirred up is used for healing purposes.

The symptoms of neuro-kundalini or pre-kundalini are somewhat similar to kundalini awakenings, but they are a lower-level expression of the energy. In my profession as a CranioSacral therapist it was incredibly common for all people, no matter their consciousness level, to twitch, release heat through their nervous system, and to move their bodies spontaneously, often in the position in which they had originally experienced trauma.

Such body-mind-spirit work operates from the premise that when the body experiences a specific trauma, such as a car crash, the direction as well as force of impact is held within the system. For example, I was in a car crash in which I was a passenger and I had both feet up on the glove box. When someone rear-ended the car behind us going forty miles an hour, I crunched forward and my left leg twisted due to the impact. During later sessions of bodywork, my nervous system released the heat; I began moving into the same position that I was in during the car crash. This had very little to do with kundalini, and more to do with releasing held trauma stored in my nervous system and body.

As a society, our nervous systems are in a state of collective disrepair, and we lack the tools and resources to process our trauma appropriately. When the nervous system begins to move from states of shock, trauma, or hyperactive dysregulation into a calmer state of being, it is not unusual to experience a release of heat and the rise of suppressed emotions. In addition, the intelligence of the body knows exactly how to move or twitch to release pent up energy.

While such expressions of energy can bring greater perspective and a certain degree of awakening, they rarely lead to the massive shifts in consciousness, experiences of bliss, greater peace or emptiness, or movement beyond basic self-interest. They often don't centralize in the spinal column or contain the positive bliss states or wide shifts in perspective that allow for an experience of liberation. However, trauma of all kinds, including neuro-kundalini states, can allow for shifts in perspective or a differing experience of daily reality to the extent that they can be an avenue for further awakening.

Kundalini Stirring & Kundalini Experiences

Kundalini is perhaps best described as a volcano located in our sacrum. In most people, it is latent. In some, it has not awakened but an occasional spark, ember, or steam arises. The volcano then goes back to its latent state, but the spark or steam arising from the volcano causes the system to consciously understand that kundalini could flow through the system.

In a kundalini-stirring experience, this volcano awakens temporarily, while sleepily and perhaps accidentally letting a bit of steam out the top. In such cases we may begin to feel sexual energy rise due to yoga practices, magical or occult rituals, or other meditative or spiritual practices. This does not mean that the volcano is active. It is more a rumbling of the volcano, with its steam and associated heat and perhaps a spark or two being let off before it goes back to latency.

Kundalini is the divine energy of creation, and our initial experiences of kundalini awakening are largely felt as sexual because of the amount of potential still in our first chakra, as well as the way the energy emerges and affects the first chakra. Our sexual energy and reproductive essence (and organs) are continually in a process of creating and maintaining unrefined spiritual energy that is naturally quite potent. We then typically use this energy for sex, reproduction, or acts of artistic creation. Many who experience kundalini stirrings as a result of spiritual, magical, or occult activities are happy to use the unrefined power of sexual energy to fuel their work.

Kundalini stirrings are temporary, and typically end quite quickly: anywhere from a moment to a few hours. There may also be an experience that lasts over a month, or a few months, with kundalini rising several times and then moving back into dormancy. It is possible to have many experiences of kundalini stirring as it is ready to awaken. This is typically experienced as heat and heightened sexual desire predominantly located in the sacrum and genitals, with an occasional sensation of heat rising in the midline, or through one of the sides of the body from the lower body.

In the case of kundalini awakening this sexual energy is refined and brought into the cerebrospinal matrix to go up the spine. This would be the actual volcano exploding, or the "snake" uncurling through the spine temporarily.

This results in a drastic shift of consciousness, spontaneous body movements (such as bowing or yogic positions that may or may not be known by the individual experiencing them), and a feeling of massive heat, or energy, rising from the first chakra. It feels like a huge electrical current, wave, or volcanic lava. There is typically a great deal of shaking, sometimes a feeling of cold releasing or circulating (depending on how kundalini flows and through which channel, as discussed in the next chapter) and an inability to attend to normal reality.

Energy flowing in through the crown and activating kundalini, rising the volcano out of dormancy, is most often experienced through *shaktipat*—being in the presence of a guru or teacher who has awakened kundalini and uses their gaze, gesture, or other methods to awaken it in their students.

While there certainly are those capable of emanating Shakti, or who have a great deal of consciousness, there are plenty of charlatans out there and people who offer shaktipat who do not have the energy awakened within themselves, or at least not to the degree of it being a catalyst to others. However, having kundalini awakened by a knowledgeable guru or teacher is an appropriate and often sought-out path for a reason. Being in the presence of a realized individual allows us to create a road map within our own system by mirroring their system. Being in the presence of someone who is quite conscious helps us recognize this same potential within ourselves.

While there are waves to kundalini, as it ebbs and flows in intensity, the evolution of spiritual intelligence and its meeting with cosmic intelligence is not a temporary thing. Nor is it something that becomes completed quickly.

A kundalini experience can be life-changing; it can be revolutionary to experience shaktipat from a realized presence. To experience lava flowing from the volcano through the system, purifying it, allowing for greater consciousness, however temporary the flow is, is life changing.

Such experiences are incredibly important. At best, we can understand them as a vital expression of creation energy emerging through the system, creating a temporary destabilization so a new ground of greater stability and consciousness can be experienced. Unfortunately we tend to pathologize such states; in any case we lack the resources in our society to tend to this destabilization process and reintegrate properly, especially if the individual experiencing such an awakening is struggling to remain functional.

A kundalini experience can lead to the permanent evolutionary process that a full kundalini awakening offers. It primes the system, allows us to understand what bliss or ecstatic states are through direct experience, and creates a purifying fire moving through the system.

In certain cases, the kundalini experience is exactly what is needed in this lifetime, whereas a permanent evolutionary process is not appropriate. Such priming can be furthered decades later, or even in the next lifetime. Kundalini permanently arising in the system is incredibly difficult to achieve, although it is often desired for good reason. We awaken to the degree that we are ready to, and those who are ready enough to experience kundalini awakenings, however temporary, have tasted something that few others do. People who have experienced any degree of awakening bring that awareness into the world, and can be of tremendous benefit to the world.

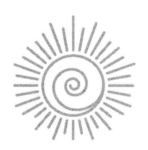

7

The First Phase of Kundalini Awakening

In the first phase of kundalini awakening, our old traumas, held emotions, and other experiences arise into conscious awareness and are released through the physical body through the fire of purification.

Such processing, especially in this stage, is always difficult. The purification is like a wildfire, burning through whatever blockages exist in the body. When we are able to handle things in a gradual manner, or if we have previously gone through basic mind-body education and healing work, we are likely to consciously work through one or two patterns simultaneously. For many of us experiencing kundalini awakening, especially abrupt awakenings in an unprepared system, this will be like hundreds or thousands of different patterns, loops, or traumas emerging at once.

This is challenging for even the most reasonable and sane soul; it can be quite difficult for us to function during the quick emotional upheavals caused by huge bursts of rage, grief, and despair, or the processing of past trauma coming into consciousness.

However, we need to understand that these upheavals destroy and reformulate our identity and unfold our consciousness. Our egos do not like change, and most of us in the first phase of kundalini awakening want to know why such material is coming up for processing, to hold on to it, identify with it, and resist the process. Change is always difficult. If we are able to surrender, and especially if we seek support to navigate such changes, we will eventually find ourselves in a place of less chaos. We start to identify less with the trauma and the identity that it has created.

What does not want us to proceed is our ego-mind, which has identified with our wounds and fracturing. If we are in a full flow state, one in which heightened consciousness begins to peek out after considerable purification has occurred, we are able to understand that we can simply move forward with our lives. We also have the energy and connections to do so.

When we have been traumatized and identify with our wounded ego-mind, we are fractured. Large parts of us are frozen, traumatized and continually reenacting whatever trauma they have experienced. Those parts of us have not caught up to our present-day consciousness, and are deeply resistant to any type of change. They want to recreate the trauma in order to find closure; we lack conscious awareness of this and so we recreate the same trauma again and again, perhaps noticing the loop (repeated behaviors) but not linking it to trauma. We get into the same relationships, have the same experiences with our boss, friends, and family.

When kundalini is in its purification fire aspect it unfreezes that held consciousness. Our trauma can arise into conscious awareness, and that aspect of ourselves that was frozen can catch up to our present-day consciousness. When we have large parts of ourselves frozen, we are devitalized. We lack energy and momentum, we are stuck, unable to meet our potential, and highly resistant. What is resistant within us stems from trauma; the frozen aspects of self are fearful of change and held within a loop of frozen circumstances. When we begin to heal, and no longer have so much of us frozen, we gain more and more vitality. No longer is our consciousness focused on what is unhealed. No longer is our life a series of repetitive loops, created chaos, and ways of seeking numbness or distractions in our lives. We begin to identify with our wholeness, health, and potential, rather than our trauma.

Due to this purification fire the first phase is filled with fluctuations of energy. We may feel extreme fatigue and need to sleep for long periods of time, and then have days or weeks when we are overflowing with energy. This is due to the body either processing trauma (which takes quite a lot of energy to accomplish) or needing deep rest to heal and rewire the nervous system. We may fluctuate between recognizing what is beyond the first phase of kundalini awakening and then being submerged in it again.

A popular term for kundalini is "spiritual power," and in the first phase this power is focused on resolving trauma through a volcanic purification process. In the second phase spiritual power feels like a stream, and the depleted energy systems of the body are revitalized.

Through the spiritual awakening process, we begin to recognize how important connection is. We realize that there is an infinite amount of energy available to us through our connections to the divine, to the earth, and to one another. If we are disconnected from the webs of life, and from the support of our communities, we only have our own energy to rely on. Kundalini awakening allows for us to connect to these webs, the sources of vitalizing energy that nurture and sustain us.

During this first phase of awakening we begin to recognize that more than our own viewpoint is valid, and we stop feeling as if the world needs to mirror our own moral and ethical compass. There is a recognition of others, and a realization of how much we ask of them. We see that the world doesn't revolve around us or our needs and traumas; we can listen to disparate viewpoints not in line with our personal biases or those of our parents. Any opening of consciousness beyond the first chakra, however small, allows us to recognize and acknowledge others.

Unfortunately there are many people involved in a process of spiritual awakening who are incredibly traumatized and seek to seal themselves off in a bubble. They say they are unable to listen to certain types of music or view certain movies, and they surround themselves only with certain types of people, typically people who have the same background, biases and ideologies as they do. This perpetuates unhealed and illusory states of disconnection, and is the diametric opposite of what the spiritual awakening process results in. Instead, the spiritual awakening process produces ease; we are better able to navigate the world and interact with the people in it. In many ways the spiritual awakening process can be described as removal of belief. Rigid beliefs and ideologies point to a lack of healing and awareness, rather than any type of higher consciousness.

Once we are beyond much of our own trauma, it is actually quite easy for compassion to develop, as we see that people are in such pain and confusion. This does not mean that we take on their viewpoint, or agree with their wounded or illusory perceptions of the world, but that we can see how people got to be who they are. We can recognize and accept people as they are; the desire to control them by wishing they would be something other than who they are lessens. In such acceptance, the need for outer approval lessens. The outer world at this point can be used as a guide to what you have left to work on; what you are still reactive to will show you the pain, loops, and held trauma you still hold within.

Other symptoms in the first phase are sexual increases and decreases, as well as automatic body movements, body locks, and shaking. This is to release held trauma from the system, as well as to create a clear passage for the oceanic flow of kundalini to move through.

In this phase, there is identification with the triple: the feminine. We begin to move from binary consciousness into nuance. We can consider one thing, its opposite, and the liminal space in between. We see how all things are impermanent, how all things change, and we recognize the feminine power of creation: death and rebirth, destruction and regeneration. We identify with the "goddess" of kundalini, and revel in her power.

We are created from the feminine, we emerge out of our mothers, we emerge out of the womb of consciousness. In heavily patriarchal societies, we revere the masculine pole, and seek to obscure or disregard our creative energy and the feminine creator. There is a long history of even very realized individuals setting up systems that do not allow spiritual education for women because of great fear of the potential of female creative power and a desire to control and restrict the spiritual realms through human ideology.

The idea that something as silly and impermanent as our physical forms has anything to do with our capacity to awaken into greater consciousness is the type of restrictive belief that always points to illusion. If anything, women have an easier time awakening, as our energetic anatomy is more internal, and our creative energy flows and cycles monthly in a way that the energetic anatomy of men does not.

In this first phase, we tend to subconsciously notice that our identity is going through a profound shift, and we tend to externalize this "death" outwardly. It is not uncommon for people to get rid of many of their belongings, to change relationships, to move, to change hair style or other identifying features.

Some of this purging is necessary; we may, for example, become acutely aware that a certain relationship or friendship is a result of karmic or unhealthy ties; once that loop has been resolved inwardly, the need for the relationship and the recreation of that loop is no longer necessary. It is also no shock for most of us to understand that this world is set up for us to grasp externally, and to seek what society determines as standards. We may decide we no longer want to participate in this. We may look around us and see what society has determined makes us valuable or worthwhile; once we recognize how much we have bought into that and how much stuff we have accumulated, we can see how unnecessary it all is.

As a spiritual worker, I frequently tell people that the first thing to do to bring new energy into your home and life is to physically clean and to donate what you have not used for a period of time. With more physical space comes more energetic opportunity. A large shift actualized in your life may be exactly what is needed. It can also be incredibly healthy to move away from people who are only causing detriment in your life.

If such urges arise, we might feel tempted to sell all of our possessions and move into a cave, to drop friendships and relationships. Sometimes that is needed. However, we may mistake a metaphorical death for a physical one. We are feeling an inward shift, an aspect of ourselves "dying"; this creates great fear, as well as an impulse to actualize this process externally. For most of us the transformation can be turned inward, refocusing the displaced energy on an internal transformative process, rather than drastically changing the external nature of our world.

Some solitude is necessary during this phase. How much depends on our individual nature and our symptoms. It is certainly important to make time to process energies and to participate in our own process, though we must be careful not to create a bubble around ourselves, which would only perpetuate the trauma-isolation cycle. The best thing we can do is ride the waves—understanding when we need solitude or when we crave connection.

Symptoms of Kundalini Awakening

The basic symptoms of kundalini awakening in this first phase are:

- Shaking or feeling of immense vibration arising from the tailbone or genitals up the midline.

- Feelings of immense heat especially around the genitals, also frequent feelings of fever in the head or body-wide.

- Spontaneous body movements and hand movements into yogic postures.

- Sexual shifts—a huge rise in sexual energy.

- Drastic shifts in consciousness—moments of transcendence, bliss states, release of identification with our chaos, projections, and wounding.

- Surges in energy—movement from highly creative, energetic states to fatigue.

- Emotional cycling, or release of huge bursts of emotional energy, especially fear.

- Spontaneous breaths and body locks—for example, the pressing of the abdomen into the spine automatically.

- Processing—spontaneous emergence of unhealed material that is rising up into consciousness to be healed.
- Digestive issues, including severe bloating.

Although there is a wide range of other symptoms that have been described in this phase, these are the ones that are being experienced by most who have kundalini awakening in their system.

However, what to look for are shifts in consciousness as a result of kundalini, not symptoms. There should be drastic shifts in perception if we are experiencing a kundalini awakening; these shifts will be absent in those in pre-kundalini states or in individuals who falsely believe they are experiencing kundalini.

There is a large reservoir of fear located within the first chakra that emerges in the first phase. Significant processing, with large emotions and trauma-related material arising all at once, indicate someone who is in the first phase, along with symptoms like large energetic flows up the midline and volcanic heat. If there is no flow of energy up the midline, which is the route or pathway for consciousness to unfold within the human form, we may be experiencing an awakening, but it is unlikely to be a kundalini awakening. There can be significant distress in this stage. So it is helpful to understand that our symptoms are byproducts of purifying fire, and a release of body-held trauma, rather than having to do with consciousness itself.

As mentioned in the previous chapter, pre-kundalini states may cause some shaking of fingers and toes, along with the mild heat from the release of trauma from the nervous system. But this is quite different from the fire, static postures, body-wide shaking, or spontaneous mudras that kundalini awakening creates. Other indicators in this initial stage are brief experiences of bliss, emptiness, or peace that drastically change consciousness. But by focusing on the transcendental experiences of kundalini awakening, we might miss identifying someone who is struggling with heavy processing, experiencing kundalini awakening in its initial stages, or simply quite stuck in their process.

The Three Bodies

How kundalini emerges within the system has a great deal to do with the predisposition of the individual. For the sake of simplicity, let us say that we have three bodies: physical, mental/emotional, and spiritual.

Picture someone who has done yoga and daily meditation for forty years. She is also a psychotherapist, has gone through psychotherapy and experienced enough bodywork to the degree that she has learned basic emotional intelligence. She has gained an adult perspective on much of the trauma she experienced in childhood and adolescence.

While the kundalini awakening process is still likely to pose difficulty for her, she is physically, mentally/emotionally, and spiritually in line and she has developed a strong nervous system in preparation for the unfolding of consciousness. Through her yogic practices she has heard of kundalini awakenings and has a mental framework for the experience. That said, the actual experience of kundalini awakening may be quite different from the intellectual or philosophical understanding she had.

She is thus primed to have a kundalini awakening where she has the framework, resources, and prior practices to work through blockages in a balanced way, and to accept both the purifying fire and kundalini awakening itself.

She may yet be surprised by the experience of consciousness shifting, or perhaps by an understanding of ancestral patterns or conscious recall of past lives but she has a stable and ready system to integrate such knowledge, or to seek out further knowledge to assist her in integrating her experiences.

Now picture someone who has never heard the word *kundalini* before. He has little awareness of the impact of diet on his body, never exercises or rarely participates in movement practices, and is emotionally unstable. He feels as if he is drowning in his life; every week is a new crisis, a new form of chaos. Beyond a yoga class or two, he has little belief in anything beyond materialist reality. He grew up believing that experiencing anything non-physical—that is, mental, emotional, or spiritual—is a sign of being unstable or even insane, and so his spiritual experiences create a huge amount of fear and denial. He is wholly oriented toward himself, unable to notice anything outside of his own life and viewpoint, or his immediate needs or wants.

Experiencing kundalini awakening will be immensely difficult for him. He already feels like he is drowning in his life and has little emotional, spiritual, or physical health or balance. Kundalini awakening is likely to feel like a giant battle, or something that will put him in a state of massive and possibly dangerous overload. He sees himself as being under attack and so he shuts down, isolates, and views the world, as well as kundalini, as a grandiose battle in which he is the eternal victim.

He is also unlikely to be able to navigate past the noise of the modern world, the types of illusions that create either the stories of immense fear or romanticization divorced from reality, in which kundalini awakening means that he will be a millionaire on a yacht with no health problems whatsoever.

He may find himself in the mental-health system or in the office of a therapist who does not understand spiritual awakenings and views any aberration from what is considered "normal" to be pathological or requiring medication. Suppression of the experience may be necessary if he goes into psychosis; this can happen if a split results from prior mental-emotional fracturing that makes it impossible for him to reconcile his daily life with emerging spiritual considerations.

In general, spiritual awakening can create symptoms that are unusual or loud, mental-emotional dysfunction, and deconstruction of the identity. This is at odds with societal expectations of normalcy, which demands emotional repression and numbness. If we awaken spiritually to any degree we will not be culturally defined as "normal," but we will have the opportunity to become what is incredibly rare in our culture: someone who has released enough trauma to be an initiated adult. However, many will find their emerging consciousness and the process of purification medicated, suppressed, or pathologized, even if such a process would lead eventually to greater stability, self-awareness, and overall consciousness.

On the other hand, it is important to note that many who believe that they are experiencing kundalini awakenings are not; it is not uncommon for those with mental-emotional imbalances to reach for spiritual labels when medication or other forms of care may be indicated. It is also significant that many may diagnose kundalini without awareness of what it is, and such a diagnosis can create more instability with a focus on the label, rather than an ability to see the process through, if it is indeed occurring.

Now, let's consider one last person. She has been meditating daily for five years. She eats a balanced diet, has participated in shamanic, spiritual, or other workshops that have given her a basic understanding of who she is and how her childhood has impacted her. She goes regularly for some type of holistic treatment. She has read Joseph Campbell and a few books on chakras. Recently she's felt as if she has had some dreams about a past life.

This is a more typical picture of someone who may begin to experience either pre-kundalini states or a kundalini awakening. While she may not be prepared for some of the shifts in identity, or the intensity of trauma processing, and will have difficulty with sleep, energy surges and fluctuations, she is nevertheless able to hold her life together. She holds down a job and tends to her family, partner, friends, and loved ones. She may go through a period of breakdown, but if she sees it through, she can re-enter the world after such a deconstruction process with greater consciousness, energy, and ability to meet the world on its terms.

Naturally she needs education, as well as practitioners who understand the process and can see it as something that is creating temporary chaos but will eventually lead to greater resiliency and consciousness. Finding that education can be difficult, but there are enough resources for those going through the first stage of kundalini awakening that she will eventually be able to find them.

Her task will be to not get stuck in her experiences, and to not identify with the emotional content and the difficulties or strangeness of the process. Much of the information regarding kundalini is about the first phase of kundalini awakening, and it tends to either glamorize or villainize the processing aspects when mental-emotional material arises, or the energetic byproducts of the process, such as body movements.

In the first phase of kundalini awakening, there is a tendency to believe that kundalini is creating the symptoms. There can also be great anger at seeing the degree of illusory knowledge in the world in regards to a topic like kundalini, or anger at going through a process like this in the modern world.

Kundalini is most simply defined as consciousness; it is our individual consciousness arising out of a latent or sleeper state. In order for us to become awake or more conscious, we need to release the traumas we have experienced, the emotions we have suppressed, the beliefs that we have created out of trauma, and all of the projections that we enact in the world. During this first phase of kundalini awakening, the fire of kundalini emerges and works its way through those barriers so we can recognize our own inherent consciousness.

If we are able to understand that the symptoms that emerge, even if they are quite extraordinary, are simply byproducts of the process, we can focus on what matters. This is what really differentiates kundalini awakenings from imbalanced or pathological states: the awakening of consciousness and its capacity for greater perspective, compassion, and stability.

The Three Types of Kundalini Awakenings

In an ideal kundalini awakening, the volcano awakens and lava rises up our midline, creating a pathway from our first chakra into our brains. We can experience severe symptoms due to it rising through the wrong channel.

There are three types of awakenings of kundalini: *pingala, ida*, and *sushumna*. If kundalini unfolds properly within the system, all three channels will eventually be opened. All three channels will go through a process of purification or stirring, and then creative potential, or consciousness, will flow through them.

These three channels form what we most commonly know as the *caduceus*. This is the central pole around which two snakes intertwine. If we consider that the "pole" is the sushumna, or spinal column, the ida and pingala wrap around this pole, bringing support as well as integrating both sides of the body with its center. Ida is associated with the left side of the body, and the lunar or feminine aspects of our nature. Pingala is associated with the right side of the body, and the solar or masculine aspects of our nature.

Both spiral around the central pole, creating an energetic gateway to the third eye, brain, and nostrils. Both ida and pingala have to do with breath as the vehicle of consciousness. This is in a very physical manner—we need oxygen to live—but also in an energetic and spiritual manner. Learning how to work with breath to navigate and control the energies within our body is deemed necessary in yogic and tantric systems to properly awaken kundalini.

Much of yogic philosophy and practice focuses on breath and its ability to activate pre-kundalini and then kundalini awakening; ida and pingala shuttle the breath through the body, activated by inhalation and exhalation. Simple practices, like alternate nostril breathing, can bring a lot to someone who has kundalini stuck in one of these channels. They can also allow us to prepare our body and nervous system so that kundalini awakening occurs gently and flows well. Such practices over many years do not appeal to a modern world so focused on attaining advanced states immediately, but they are the best route to awakening if done with a competent teacher.

The entirety of this "highway," or sushumna, ida, and pingala, together, physically as well as spiritually, have to do with how our nervous system is functioning. This highway activates and rewires in a process like kundalini. It is not unusual to see images of DNA (the "spiral" of ida, pingala, and sushumna) when this process is occurring.

Ideally we would do years or even decades (if not lifetimes) of preparatory practices for kundalini to awaken in our systems, much of that time devoted to working with the breath and its capacity to flow and unblock differentiated energy, and then kundalini.

Some of us may have had kundalini awaken in our systems without understanding the significance of such practices. The automatic stopping or locking of the breath in specific parts of the body to propel kundalini fire through the system will be confusing for anyone who does not have an understanding that such experiences parallel high yogic practices.

Even if we have a background in yoga, or have a knowledgeable teacher, much of the spiritual and in-depth knowledge of such structures is never related, either due to ignorance or because most yoga studios and teachers must understandably focus on beginners, and beginners' courses, to pay the rent.

Many modern-day spiritual practices are intended to create catharsis or loud spiritual experiences to convince the spiritually orphaned individual that there are spiritual realms or energies outside of our materialist reality. Finding a teacher who has traversed the path to find stability and clarity, and who recognizes the worth of gradual, foundational practices with something like breathwork, is key. Breathwork and other spiritual practices focused on creating catharsis, or loud spiritual experiences, can be detrimental to individuals already involved with what can be a chaotic spiritual experience; we may also realize that something loud or explosive is not needed to convince us of spiritual reality, or we may be beyond needing an adrenaline rush through spiritual interface.

Kundalini should unfold through the spinal column and midline of the body—the sushumna. This is how it properly uncurls, how the snake properly rises and pierces through the chakras, leading to consciousness unfolding within the system. If it rises through pingala first, severe difficulties can emerge.

Perhaps the most famous tale of kundalini awakening through pingala (the channel on the right) is Gopi Krishna. He went through incredibly difficult symptoms and experiences. While I recommend his book (in the further reading section) his is a tale of how kundalini can go quite wrong through incorrect meditation methods and create severe symptoms that persist over a long time. These may include severe heat, issues on the right side of the body, the emergence of trauma that cannot be purified correctly, and a perpetuation and heightening of mental-emotional imbalances.

In our Western world we revere the masculine. We hunger after spirituality for its peak experiences; we need something large, explosive, and chaotic to either distract us from our lives or to show us that something exists beyond scientific materialist reality. We go to military style workshop retreats that are incredibly intensive and create sleep deprivation for weeks, we take plant medicines not revering their inherent divinity but seeking a high, we go towards intense or advanced practices without establishing a foundation first.

We are also incredibly traumatized, and accustomed to forceful, cathartic, purging, or traumatizing experiences in our lives. We lack emotional intelligence, and look to suppress any and all emotions, to anesthetize them, to forcibly transmute them, especially the ones that we have deemed "bad," leading to generations of individuals with massive backlogs of anger, fear, apathy, depression, and grief. We lack nurturing, an appreciation for silence, gentleness, or compassion for ourselves and others. We lack self-love. For this reason, we reach for practices that involve self-flagellation. Our self-obsession guides our spiritual searches, which often result in further self-obsession rather than any type of awakening or ability to see beyond our individual experiences of this world.

Kundalini awakenings emerge through pingala because hard, fast, cathartic, or incorrect practices open up the channel associated with such an imbalance. There may also be a blockage in the first chakra significant enough that kundalini is unable to flow upward, and so it utilizes pingala as a way to let off steam, or lava, from that volcano.

This is complicated by the fact that ida and pingala are smaller channels than sushumna. Any type of awakening is meant to be in conjunction with the central channel to ensure proper balance and regulation, as well as to properly unfold consciousness through the system.

If we return to the idea of kundalini awakening being like a dormant volcano, we also need to understand that many who are experiencing kundalini awakenings are not going through a process of unfolding consciousness; that dormant volcano is either sending steam or has flung out a glob of lava randomly. This can go up pingala and get stuck in the pingala channel, but it does not represent a full awakening of the system, or even kundalini awakening and arising through the channel. This will create symptoms and exacerbate mental-emotional or physical nervous system issues, but it isn't a purifying fire. There is not enough lava or steam to clear the blocks out of the system.

In severe states, individuals in this group lack even the most basic compassion and regard for human beings, and will express beliefs that run counter to anything that a grounded, realized individual would say or believe.

There are an unfortunate number of spiritual teachers and seekers in the modern world who are simply not healthy or who are steeped in illusion. Such teachers can be seen as gatekeepers; moving beyond their illusory or imbalanced wisdom is an initiation beyond the gate that such a teacher provides. Such teachers are needed in this world, as they free up more experienced and knowledgeable teachers to work with sincere seekers looking for clarity and evolution.

Even a little bit of conscious awareness beyond the first chakra allows us to recognize others around us, to feel compassion for their pain, and to see their perspective, even if it is dissimilar to our own. Individuals still locked in the first chakra state of awareness, even with pingala awakened, lack this regard and point to themselves. They often believe that they have experienced advanced states of consciousness, which has only served for them to judge and have contempt for the rest of humanity while believing themselves to be superior and separate. If we have even a brief glimpse of the cosmos, or perspective beyond our ego-mind, we realize our basic connectivity and recognize how small we are in the grand scheme of things. Any experience of divinity releases the illusion that we are superior in any way, and the ego and its desire for specialness, control, knowing, and separation will be revealed as false.

Consciousness unfolding requires our participation and significant effort. Those who have not moved beyond the first chakra will believe that they have achieved advanced states with little to no effort, and are not yet at a point where they are willing or able to participate in their own evolution.

Others who experience pingala awakening are those who do so momentarily through a variety of spiritual practices, or through readiness of their system. Things like headaches, nasal issues, and pains on the right side of the body emerge as a result. However, the emergence of symptoms like these do not point to awakening unless the consciousness of the individual is undergoing change; this widened viewpoint, and the movement beyond basic selfishness, and not the symptoms, are what to look for in any type of awakening.

Other individuals who have pingala awakenings are a result of sudden awakenings with no prior preparation of their systems or who practice intensive or catharsis-related spiritual activities, similar to extreme sports. They may also be mentally-emotionally imbalanced or traumatized to the extent that they have an immense amount of material at their first chakra; kundalini emerging there is like an ocean hitting a wall: it will find another outlet, such as pingala, for some of the emerging energy to flow.

These individuals tend to have the worst and most nightmare-ish of kundalini awakening experiences. They will associate kundalini awakening with the traumatized material that is attempting to emerge, or may turn to numbing mechanisms, such as drug use, to neglect what is happening inwardly. Substance use and abuse is prevalent on the spiritual path, as the overwhelm that such an experience creates, as well as the wear and tear of the continual destabilization and reformation of the personality (ego) is difficult to manage for even the most stable of souls.

Only by returning to our first chakra, putting forwards some effort to participate in our own evolution, reaching out for support, and by not falling victim to any ego traps, will we find kundalini awakening and unfolding through the sushumna in a proper manner. This typically requires outer support, as we may create illusions that we do not need support to continue a lack of clarity or to perpetuate trauma loops.

Awakening first in ida is fairly rare. Symptoms include feeling cold or shivers throughout the system. Ida is our lunar, feminine side; it holds our emotions and is responsible for our hormonal and endocrine balance. Ida is associated with our deeply held emotions, our *yin* emotions such as deep grief, despair, and trauma to the parasympathetic system; this creates deep freeze instead of the fight or flight that is associated with nervous system overload.

Symptoms such as left leg stiffness and dysfunction are commonly experienced by those experiencing kundalini awakenings, which seemingly have a link to ida; these symptoms lessen with activation of the channel in conjunction with sushumna and pingala.

Symptoms emerging in pingala tend towards loud expressions: huge shaking, fear, manic states, delusional states, and expression of mental-emotional symptoms that render the person incapable of functioning in their lives. Those who experience ida awakenings are more internal already, and more open to receiving treatment, to educating themselves, as well as to noticing that something is off balance within their systems. Both ida and pingala awakenings also have symptoms with pressure in the third eye, as well as nasal issues, as that is where those channels run. If there is a glob of kundalini fire that has made its way into those systems, we may be well aware of where that glob is; the termination point of those channels—the nostrils and third eye—tend to be where people experience the greatest sensation.

A wide range of pain disorders—migraines and headaches, nervous system problems, immune issues, functional disorders (ones that do not show up on a test but are typically labeled by a constellation of different symptoms)—may be a result of kundalini arising through ida and pingala. Careful differentiation, focus on prior trauma, and soothing the nervous system are indicated first for any of these issues, whether they are a result of kundalini awakening or not.

It is all too easy to put a whole list of symptoms and disorders that are currently mysterious or dismissed by modern medicine onto kundalini awakening. Despite how kundalini starts or arises, a focus on self-healing and trauma care is necessary. Without the symptoms of consciousness expansion and unfolding, purification fire and processing of what is held in the system, and experiences of shaking, heat, or energetic rising up the midline, it is highly unlikely to be kundalini awakening.

The First Stage and Symptoms

We may be spiritually awakening in a variety of ways, but without energy moving through the midline resulting in huge shifts in consciousness, it is unlikely to be a kundalini awakening. Paramahansa Yogananda called the spinal cord and the brain "the altar to God"; it is evident through a wide variety of spiritual, occult, and religious disciplines that without spiritual energy emerging through the midline, consciousness fails to evolve to any significant degree.

If we again return to our understanding of the three "bodies"—physical, mental/emotional, and spiritual—the symptoms we experience are going to be a direct result of any imbalance or weakness in one of those bodies.

The snake that is unfolding (a traditional understanding of the term "kundalini" would be more in line with the word "curl") and rising up the midline can be thought of as poisonous, and as it pierces each chakra, it releases what is held within that section of the body. When it then rises beyond the chakra, it is no longer "poisonous" to that chakra or area of the body as it moves to pierce a new chakra.

As the snake uncurls three and a half times, rising and straightening through the system, the purification process is intense, volcanic, and demanding, as old traumas and blockages rise into consciousness for resolution. The snake fully rising and straightening allows the purification cycle to complete; we attain self-realization, and individual consciousness meets cosmic consciousness. During the first phase, the purification is intense, but it abates in the second phase of kundalini when energetic flows are experienced that are more watery, rather than fiery in nature.

We can have many experiences of energy surges above the head. In some cases this is differentiated energy, and for others this will be like a volcanic explosion of kundalini creating a pathway and purging a great deal of material from the physical form in a short period of time.

There is a lot of emphasis on the automatic body movements that are created in the kundalini awakening process. If we consider our meridians (channels and/or nadis) to be a series of pipes, the flow of consciousness through them will allow for release of what is stuck in those pipes (trauma and personal history in this first stage). Differentiated energy already has difficulty moving through the joints and curves of the human body; the pre-kundalini awakening process begins to create larger pipes so that differentiated energy and then kundalini can flow through.

Consciousness itself (kundalini) is a larger flow, and has even greater difficulty moving through the joints and curves of the human form. There is the need for even larger and wider pipes so that kundalini can flow through. If there is a large flow of kundalini, it will be like a waterfall flowing through our system. The way that we are currently organized within gravity (how we stand, sit, use our physical form) may mean that kundalini can simply flow through; it may also create an immense amount of pain, like a huge ocean current slamming against a rock.

The shaking, body movements, and other automatic movements, including body locks (where the body pauses and holds breath quite severely, often felt in this phase in the perineum pulsation as well as the diaphragm) are to open up the physical form to allow this flow through, as well as to create new "pipes" to allow greater and greater flows of kundalini through the body. The release of trauma and the influx of greater flows of spiritual energy can also create shifts in vibration and consciousness, with effects of shaking, cold, heat, or trauma releasing from the system as a result.

Digestion, Sleep, and Energy Fluctuations

The fire that releases impurities, such as held emotions, can cause significant digestive distress. Our digestive tract is a series of tubes that get filled with unprocessed food as well as unprocessed emotions, thoughts, and trauma.

But there is also a process that is best understood as a *rerouting of the digestive fire*. In unawakened states, we are intended to digest not only physical food but also our emotions and thoughts. If we are in a state of overwhelm, exhaustion, or already struggling with suppressed emotions, we will be unable to fully process the nature of our days, or our lives. This is especially true if we do not enter states of true rest, or non-doing, in which our nervous system gets a chance to move from being turned on to an off position.

Throughout our lives we naturally are intended to enter states of "rest and digest" to resolve what goes on in our lives. However, in the modern world most of our nervous systems are in such a state of disarray that many of us exist in a state of continual panic, unable to process even the simplest aspects of our day, let alone the big disruptions or traumas.

In the kundalini awakening process, the nature of heavy processing requires a great deal of "digestion" as traumas held by the system arise all at once into consciousness. This is done through the digestive tract, which not only digests physically but also energetically.

During the first phase of rerouting of the digestive fire, the digestive system is no longer able to function. We may go through periods of being able to eat only very small meals, simple meals, or specific foods. We naturally have a "fire" that is intended in normal capacity to "heat" the material coming in to assimilate and digest it. When kundalini awakens, this same mechanism becomes inflamed and shuts down in order to allow for greater processing. Our processing is focused on spiritual information, which limits the ability to process other input, such as food.

During the second phase of rerouting, a rewiring process begins. This is similar to an electrician shutting off the fuse box and all of the lights in the house in order to rewire the house. The abdomen is a considerable reservoir of spiritual energy. It is not only the energy derived from the food that we eat, and the breath that we cycle through our bodies, but also the fire that forms the basis of our entire energetic system, known in Chinese medicine as *ming men*. The *ming men* is where undifferentiated energies (not yet polarized into female and male qualities) are stored. It is the root of our essence and of the energies that have been passed down to us through heredity.

If you look at realized individuals, they typically have something of a pot belly. It is not unusual for people experiencing kundalini awakenings to go through periods in which their abdomens look like they are nine months pregnant. The abdomen is rewiring, or opening, to be able to accept the full flow of kundalini; it also allows for greater breath, leading to the eventual downflow of grace. The rerouting of the digestive fire facilitates both drastic healing and purification of the system; it also creates the potential for an important alchemical process in which our *yin* (female) and *yang* (masculine) energies converge within the body.

In the third phase of rerouting, the cutting of the abdominal knot creates the capacity for the original fire of the body, the *ming men*, to create and store undifferentiated spiritual energy within the human body.

The digestive fire takes considerable time to reroute, and only completes in the third phase, if it does complete. The completion of this cycle is only evident in highly realized individuals who have fully awakened kundalini within their systems.

It is typical for people experiencing kundalini awakenings in the first phase to have to completely change their diet, to go through periods of limited diets, or to discover that with heightened energy, their need for food intake decreases.

With the eventual full flow of kundalini as it cycles to the brain and into the heart center in the third phase, the digestive issues lessen. Realistically, specific dietary measures and significant digestive dysfunction are permanent for even the most realized of individuals. Hypothetically, the digestive issues that arise in kundalini awakenings would cease with the complete rooting of undifferentiated spiritual energies within the abdomen, but that is something that very few individuals in history have attained.

The change in sleep patterns is something that affects many people in the first phase of kundalini awakening. Somnolence, or the desire to sleep for longer periods, cycling with periods of insomnia, are quite common. When we are asleep we are able to deeply process, to restore and renew, without the conscious mind (ego) interfering. We are able to have greater access to our subconscious, to the symbols and myths that are a bridge between our spiritual and psychological nature. We also may begin to have spiritual dreams in this phase, dreaming that we are interacting with teachers or having other transpersonal experiences.

This can easily turn into insomnia, periods of heightened creativity, heightened sexuality, or even mania. The body burns feverishly during periods like this. We may experience depression that accompanies the desire for lengthy sleep, or anxiety that accompanies the heightened energetic process; what distinguishes a spiritual awakening from clinical depression or bipolar states is the resolution of issues and the expansion of consciousness. With particularly difficult sleep patterns or dramatic cycling of personal energy, it is often helpful to see if kundalini energy is routing through pingala instead of sushumna. This creates cycling and switching back and forth of energy, but without any of the resolution, expanded consciousness, or increased ability to meet the world that the fire going through the sushumna creates.

We tend to judge ourselves with regards to what is considered societally appropriate or psychologically normal in terms of sleep and energy. Kundalini awakening is beyond the context of normalcy, or of typical psychological considerations; if we attend to our bodies we can accept that they need to sleep for twelve hours a few nights in a row, or even for a few weeks.

We also can begin to use periods of heightened energy and creativity to get things done, knowing that the crest of the wave and the expansion of our system is likely to retract at some point. Once we are no longer in a state of total fear or overwhelm, we can ride such waves.

Release of the Old: Death and Rebirth

When kundalini awakens and our individual consciousness meets cosmic consciousness, we realize the truth of our eternal nature. We see that what we have attended to our entire lives has been noise and chaos and illusion. We step back into witnessing, emptiness, peace, silence, or sometimes bliss: a first recognition of our authentic nature.

This shift is sometimes referred to as "ego death": the destruction of identity, and the reformulation of a new identity. With an ego death experience, we can submerge into oneness, emptiness, feelings of flow, joy, bliss, or complete dissolution.

The spiritual awakening process leads us to experience oneness. The individual ego refines itself, goes though death and rebirth many times as consciousness expands into understanding oneness. Our perspective shifts to being a witness to what is false, to what blocks us from the full potential of our individual consciousness. Paradoxically, it is also about discovering the cosmic "I." The merging of individual consciousness with cosmic consciousness is not a state of emptiness, but the realization of divine individual purpose. It is an understanding of ourselves as a drop in the ocean and the entirety of the ocean simultaneously. It is an expansion and contraction process, a state where oneness and individuation are experienced simultaneously.

My Experiences of the First Stage

The first stage of kundalini awakening for me lasted about eight years. Full-fledged symptoms emerged when I was twenty-three; my initial reaction was one of fear, shock, and disbelief.

This fear is pretty typical for people in this first stage. Our first chakra is the storehouse of fear, and when kundalini first emerged, it did so quite violently in me. I have had strange experiences since I was a child, but the symptoms and experiences I had during this time were far removed from any physical or psychological process that I recognized. This perpetuated unhealed myths that there was something terribly wrong with me.

My awakening first began in the sushumna and the first chakra but like many modern experiencers who did not have prior preparation or a decent teacher, it quickly rerouted to pingala. I had experienced migraines since I was a teenager and can recognize now that kundalini had begun to awaken; combined with my sensitivities this had launched a bit of "lava" occasionally into the pingala channel starting in my early teens. But my awakening this time was pure fire.

During this period my pulse went from being in the low 70s to the high 90s, or even occasionally in the low 100s. I knew this because I was in my initial stages of acupuncture education, in which we took our pulses quite regularly.

While I was no stranger to existential depression and deep feeling, I realized that in order to meet the world I had shoved most of what I felt deeply within. We do not reward depth of feeling or existential questioning kindly in this world, and I had learned from an early age that my thoughts, as well as what I was experiencing, were not something to express outwardly.

I really struggled with the initial emotional fluctuations. I didn't understand the huge wellspring of rage and grief that emerged. So many experiences and memories were coming up simultaneously that I couldn't differentiate them all. As of yet I had no education about the impact of past lives or ancestors or anything beyond typical psychology and so when I began to have dreams and realizations that went beyond those boundaries, I went through long periods of fear and denial in regards to what I was experiencing.

All this was incredibly confusing to me, as was most of this initial process; I didn't understand that my body was attempting to process what was within me. I was also incredibly resistant. I felt that kundalini was victimizing me, that I was in a great battle with it, one that I was not winning.

Most difficult during the first phase were my digestive issues. I spent the better part of two years eating rice, or sometimes avocados or cooked vegetables. During the initial part of my process I was unable to digest dairy, meat, spice, nightshades, or complex foods (more than a few ingredients). They would cause me to either vomit or experience extreme digestive distress to the point that I would need fluids or even emergency room care. I went through periods when I felt large shaking going up my midline, which brought dizziness and nausea; there was nothing I could do but sit quietly and wait for this to pass.

I went through all sorts of tests for both my migraines and digestive issues but nothing was ever found. Beyond basic potassium issues from acute distress, or small or borderline hormonal changes, there were few answers for me through allopathic medicine, or even through naturopathic care. Instead of this creating relief, it filled me with anger. I was having such severe symptoms and I wanted them named and labeled and fixed. Even when I fully believed that I was in fact experiencing a kundalini awakening, I was still hopeful that many of my more painful and disruptive experiences would be explained through mechanistic means.

One of the largest patterns that came up for me was ancestral healing. I had participated in therapy as a child and teenager. As someone who was adopted at the age of two and a half, my early childhood experiences were supposedly at the root of any and all of my problems. I always felt that there was something deeper than that, and I resented having to go to counselors, especially when it took me away from something like music class.

I had a friend who once expressed this sentiment quite a bit better than I could. He was in a plane crash when he was ten years old in which he lost his mother and sister; every therapist or bodyworker he went to, upon hearing this, would nod knowingly and want to focus on that experience. Yet he felt that even if that trauma was the root of 97 percent of his issues, the other three percent could use some attending to.

Certainly early childhood and any adolescent trauma needs to be looked at and healed. But throughout my life I had a palpable sense of grief and fear, and I had dreams that pointed to experiences that felt linked to me yet were not my own.

I also felt strangely displaced and uprooted. My parents never hid the fact that I was adopted, and at age twelve my mother pulled out the sheet of paper that listed the basic facts of what was known about me. On the list were the countries of my heritage: Yugoslavia, Serbo-Croatia, Czechoslovakia, with a bit of Irish thrown in. My mother laughed and said that it made sense—none of the countries that I was from existed anymore.

I didn't really think about this for many years. But later I started to understand the patterns that came from those ancestors: the sort of toughness where I could be in extreme pain or break a leg and still continue, fears around lack of food, fear that I experienced of my home being broken into at night, and immense feelings of grief, displacement, and despair. My mother had tuned into another factor: I was often in existential types of questioning. During the first phase, I found the right resources and educated myself, and the heaviness began to lift.

I recognize now that I was attracted to CranioSacral therapy because it allowed me to process in a body-focused way the energetic blockages in my sushumna, thus freeing kundalini to unfold correctly. Instead of processing things alone, my education and the workshops that I attended gave me a huge amount of treatment and support during this decade. There is no way to express how grateful I am for the support I received from so many caring and compassionate individuals during this period of my life.

Over time, the drastic heat began to wane, to flow and ebb. I began to experience huge shudders as well as shaking up my spine. I experienced drastic shifts in consciousness, in which I went into ecstatic states and felt past patterns and aspects of identity release. Such states were overwhelming, and created huge outpourings of emotions. Each time I experienced an ecstatic state, I would feel dark, disconnected, and moody for days or weeks after. Then the depressive state would lift, and I would realize how my consciousness had expanded, my perceptions changed, and my body's energy flowed more freely.

I learned that my body movements were largely to force energy past blockages and through the joints and crevices of my body. I began doing yoga. I saw that part of the reason my process was so difficult was that my physical body was severely out of balance. By consciously participating in my own embodiment process, I started to be able to dance, to shake, to twist and do yoga positions while working with kundalini. This was very different from feeling like a violating power was forcing me to do such things.

As I moved into the second stage, I had a near-death experience that drastically changed my outlook and identity.

This happened five years in, and after that I began to have increasing spiritual experiences. This did not happen right away; I spent my last year of formalized education (getting my master's degree in Chinese medicine) in a state of shock. This was paired with considerable fatigue and an inability to process such an abrupt change. The near-death experience severed the knot of the abdominal chakra for me, and I struggled to integrate the perspective and consciousness shifts, especially as I was supposed to be focused on completing coursework and clinical rotations as well as board exams for my degree.

I have found that many people need a near-death experience to sever this knot. From my vantage point now I can see that my near-death experience released a lot of unprocessed material, especially surrounding death. Having such an experience allowed me to move beyond identifying with my physical form. That said, although the experience may have been necessary at the time to move me beyond this knot, I do think now that this shift could have been enacted on a more metaphorical, rather than a physical, level.

While I was still working with the sheaths in my first, second, and third chakras, kundalini began focusing on my solar plexus, heart, and throat. I experienced a certain lightness overall, as well as improved capacity to function, as the second curl began to unfold.

I realized with clarity how selfish my former self had been, and how immersed in self-obsession most people in the world were. This was a harsh thing for me to see within myself, and a big part of the second stage for me involved reconciling the perpetrator aspects of me, the past selves who were less conscious. I felt a lot of grief for my less conscious selves, as well as grief for humanity.

Through this stage the word *truth* guided me, and at a certain point I realized that it was time to surrender that word, though it had successfully allowed me to move beyond using the spiritual path to fuel further self-obsession.

Healing Suggestions for the First Stage

In a general sense I suggest working on providing stability and strengthening the "body" that you are weakest in: the physical body, mental-emotional body, or the spiritual body. For those of you who are basically functional, I recommend volunteering, learning how to properly meditate, doing physical exercise, as well as practicing self-inquiry and healing work.

This means light to moderate exercise, or even a simple daily walk, for those who are disembodied, disassociated, or lack physical health. Working with the physical form creates a body that is able to handle the rewiring process and shifts that occur much better than one that lacks physical health. I recommend a gradual method of physical exercise and strengthening the body. For example, if you have not gotten off of the couch and have been in crisis for the last two weeks, an hour of yoga is probably not indicated. But a walk around the block might be. If there is a reasonable level of health, start with thirty minutes a day of movement-based exercise.

If you are in crisis, it is a good idea to stop any spiritual activity: meditating, reading spiritual books, going to workshops or participating in online groups. While many individuals in online groups are well meaning, they often lack information, clarity or psychological stability. A focus on receiving trauma care is indicated, as is working with a grounded teacher or healer who can assist you in processing.

If there is stability of the mental-emotional body, you may practice daily meditation and/or self-inquiry, such as working with my book, *The Body Deva*.

Volunteering

I jokingly refer to the first phase of kundalini awakening as *getting over yourself*. It is quite easy in the modern world to think that spiritual awakening is about furthering self-obsession or even perpetuating illusion or wounding patterns. It is also quite easy if we lack balance and perspective in our lives to separate or disassociate from the world.

The purpose of the spiritual path can be described as many things. The reference to *getting over yourself* is something of a joke to state that this phase brings you beyond the sort of chaos and noise that you once involved yourself in; it also encourages you to consider how you may be of benefit to the world, instead of simply taking what you can from it.

One of the things that happens in this first phase is a retraction of energy. This happens to any of us when we are in pain. We must tend to ourselves to ensure our survival. What can happen in this retraction is that symptoms are exacerbated, and we just sit mired in our own chaos, rather than opening our eyes to the world around us.

Volunteering is a great way to ensure that you move beyond self-obsession and begin to turn your energy outward again. Being of benefit to others changes your mood. For centuries being of service, from karma yoga to the concept of being a *mensch*, has been proposed as a way to become more conscious.

Ideally, to experience the spiritual awakening benefits of volunteering, you would volunteer out of sincere, heartfelt desire to help your fellow human being—not because society dictates that is what good people do or because you view yourself as helping lesser beings. But even if you start grumbling and not feeling well and just doing volunteer work because there is a glimmer of hope that it might make you feel a bit better, you are still being of benefit to the world; and in that capacity, your energy again begins cycling. You are connecting to the world in a way that inspires health.

Trauma Healing and Bodywork

The first thing to do when experiencing a kundalini awakening is to focus on healing trauma patterns. That way we participate in the purifying fire of the first phase. If we are seeing through the eyes of trauma, we have a restricted view of the world that lacks adult consciousness. Healing brings us into present, full, and flowing consciousness.

If we are drowning or treading water in our lives we need support. Working with healers can help us work through larger blocks, see our blind spots, and make sure we are not misleading ourselves or veering into illusion.

The parts of ourselves that are the most broken, those from the earliest stages (such as infancy or in utero) cannot be healed alone. Those patterns are too primary, and need to be witnessed by someone who is compassionate and stable.

Our larger patterns have that same need. They are stuck in the same story; they need to tell their story and to have their needs met to find closure. We can do some of this for ourselves, but if we are in overwhelm, unstable or unable to function, we need healers as a guiding force. We also may have blind spots to our largest wounds, and an outer perspective is required to help us come into conscious awareness of them.

Even for the most stable of individuals, this phase is incredibly difficult and support is indicated. There is no need to suffer alone, and there are plenty of competent individuals that can help us process our trauma.

Solitude and Nature

Nature is typically the first thing that we feel truly comfortable connecting to, and is the easiest access point we have to the divine. If we have had difficult experiences with people we may not wish to connect to them or feel safe in receiving nurturing from them. We may not fully trust ourselves yet to keep ourselves safe.

We are intended to connect. It is how we stay healthy; it is how we stay sane. One of the largest reasons that there is so much trauma in the modern world is that we are so disconnected. Most of us are crying out for nurturing and connection. Learning to connect to nature, rely on it, brings a sense of release and stability. In nature we can experience divinity.

If possible, I suggest that you seek solitude for at least three consecutive days every six months as long as you are in this stage. You might sit in a cabin or camp or go someplace where you can sit in silence for most of the day and allow processing to occur. Ideally you will attune your senses to the natural world—the darkest of darks, the vibrancy of the dawn.

If you are in any way suicidal or feel like you are drowning in your life, this is not the time for solitude, but for human connection. To go into solitude I suggest having reasonable physical as well as emotional stability. Also be in a place where you can reach out to friends or family if something arises that needs to be witnessed, or a lonely or despairing aspect of you emerges.

Dancing and Moving with Kundalini

If we understand kundalini to be the forced flow of consciousness through the system, and understand that such flows have difficulty moving through the joints and crevices of the body, we can realize much of the purpose for spontaneous movements. These movements are exacerbated by the rewiring or creation of new pipes, or the widening of pipes in the system so that qi (differentiated energy) and then kundalini can flow.

Such movements can be terrifying for people in this stage. Shaking and body movements release held trauma, and in this stage we are immersed in the fear being released by the first chakra. There may also be understandable concerns for safety as well as significant trauma that is created through the process itself, or by feeling that we are lacking control of the physical form.

Starting to work with kundalini by dancing or doing yoga can alleviate symptoms dramatically, and it can significantly cut down on the fear response. If you do not have a background in yoga or other movement exercises (such as qi gong or tai chi) seek out a basic course of instruction with an established teacher. However, what tends to be helpful in this phase is not having a static course of instruction but moving the body in conjunction with the flow of consciousness.

This means establishing safety (a room with no sharp objects and ideally a bit of space for a yoga mat), listening to intuition and dancing or moving in ways that allow kundalini to flow. That way you feel like an active participant in the process. However, at this phase, slow and gentle movement is better than wild and fast. Gentle moving postures, static body postures and hand gestures will naturally and intuitively happen to assist kundalini cycling.

Sexual Activity

It is typically recommended that during this period people refrain from sexual activity. This is because kundalini can be many things, most of which have to do with creation energy: sexual energy, essence, orgasmic energy. Through the process of kundalini awakening we are continually tapping into this creation energy and dying and birthing ourselves along the pathway of consciousness.

Our sexual energy, even in its raw and unrefined form, is powerful. During the kundalini awakening process, the unrefined sexual essence is refined and transmitted up the spine. If this energy is released through the sexual act or masturbation, the unrefined energy is released downward.

I have known some individuals with blocks in their first chakra who have experienced such a fierce kundalini awakening that they are unable to function because their sex drive is so high. I have had reported to me such heat in this area that the perineum and genitals become inflamed (not infected), burning through the cloth in the seat of the pants, and an inability to attend to anything else in life. These individuals will release this energy downward when it builds up too high as a way to lessen discomfort.

I find that most people will naturally stop having sex for a period of time if they are experiencing a kundalini awakening. This allows the sexual essence to be transformed and kundalini to reach the brain.

Questions for Self-Enquiry

By far the biggest danger on the spiritual path is using it to foster illusions out of trauma. By questioning yourself, you can move beyond this, or begin to see where your needs for healing lie. The following questions can be utilized to move beyond common illusions in the first phase.

Separating or connecting?

There is a fair amount of nuance to this question. If we believe that we "see no color" or that "we are all on the same level and have equal things to offer," this lacks any type of nuance. Our diversity, our differences, our unique expression of the elements is to be celebrated. We all have varying levels of intelligence, experience, study, skill, consciousness, and aptitude. Noting our differences without being motivated by questions of superiority/inferiority (see below) represents clear and discriminating seeing. In differentiated reality, we are not all the same and do not all have the same aptitude, knowledge, skills, or intellect.

People who have not experienced oneness do not understand this paradox; we are one *and* different. We inhabit several levels of reality simultaneously. On one level we are all one, but on the physical plane we are not. I sometimes joke to people who believe that oneness means we have no differences, or should not judge, and ask them if they would have surgery from someone who has not been to medical school, or ask them to give me their keys, wallet, purse, car, or credit card. If we are all one, I would like to experience oneness with their credit card!

We can use this question to see how aspects of our consciousness have frozen and fractured. By identifying or asking if something that you believe is *connecting you to yourself* or *separating you from yourself (and the world)* you can cut through a lot of trauma-based illusion and see what lies within that could use healing. Our trauma always disconnects us from ourselves and the world, while consciousness connects us to ourselves and the world.

Superior or inferior?

If we are acting from our wounds rather than what is healed within us, many of our actions will come from either feeling inferior or needing to be seen as superior. Sometimes both emerge simultaneously. It can be easy to see that those who constantly need to judge or put down other individuals often feel unhealed and unworthy themselves.

The superiority-inferiority loop is our most basic loop (repeated pattern emerging from trauma); we repeat it again and again. We point to others who are false, or we continually create illusions that we are superior. Anyone who has moved beyond the first phase of kundalini awakening has broken through this loop and can see how much time and energy people spend enacting it in the outer world. When this loop does emerge for us we can use it to heal the feelings of inferiority that are at the root of it. We can see how the people we are pointing to in the outer world are unrealized aspects of ourselves, and we can heal our projections.

Questioning whether you are motivated by feeling superior or inferior lets you reassess your actions and thoughts and see through false beliefs. What is healed and realized within us does not need to feel superior or inferior. There may be things that we are not good at; we may recognize others or ourselves at varying stages of development in our skills, tools, knowledge, and consciousness. That is quite different from feeling superior or inferior to somebody else; it is more like noting that they can build a house, while you cannot hammer a nail straight.

What age am I?

When we wish to speak or take action, we can question what age is speaking or wishes to act. For example, you may realize that your teenage self wants to get into a fight; then you can remember that you are forty-seven, not a teenager, and you have better things to do. You can also begin to see what ages dominate your beliefs and create the most blockages in your life.

What motivates me in this instance?

Questioning our basic motivations is always helpful. If we are doing something that does not benefit or support another, we may be doing it out of boredom or to externalize our feelings. Or we may be trying to dump energy on someone or vampirisize their energy. Coming to terms with our basic motivations can show us what needs healing within; stopping ourselves when we are not seeking to be of benefit or cannot be compassionate will decrease the amount of drama in our lives.

Is this a metaphorical or physical death?

Our minds lack the ability to differentiate between physical and metaphorical dying. Great fear emerges at any type of change in this stage. By questioning whether it is a metaphorical or physical death, we can realize that it is likely a metaphorical death, and the nervous system and mental-emotional body can release some of its fear.

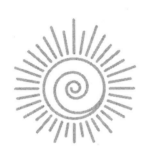

8

The Second Phase of Kundalini Awakening

During the second phase of kundalini the spiritual heart begins to open and we recognize ourselves as consciousness. While there is still personal material to attend to, the focus has moved away from the self and into considering societal, historical, cultural, and other forms of conditioning.

The solar plexus, heart, throat, and third eye chakras open in this phase. The first stages of enlightenment and flows of heightened consciousness begin to be experienced on a continual basis, expressed as inner music, spontaneous vocalization, witnessing of inner deities, and large creative flows, as well as an experience of grace, or downward flow.

In the previous stage, we identify as someone experiencing kundalini. In the second stage, we understand kundalini as consciousness itself. We go through heightened states as well as vibration and pulsation and we have a direct experience of infinity.

Our experiences shift away from the purifying fire and into a sense of water, or flow, within. While there will still be some purification heat, the focus is now on creating a pathway of clear or golden light through the midline, allowing for self-realization to occur.

Other symptoms include:

- Movement past societal and other forms of conditioning
- Static and devotional postures, ecstatic dancing
- Throat contractions and tongue thrusting
- Realization of impact of time, ability to see through time, dimensions, and existence in multiple layers of reality simultaneously
- Acceptance that what is in the world is also within the self
- Change in breath, long retention of automatic breaths

- Opening of the portals of the head (senses: hearing of divine music, smells, synesthesia; headaches and sinus issues)
- Acceptance of all aspects of self, including emotions
- Processing of deeper karma, self as persecutor
- Processing of atavistic instincts and self-hatred
- Realization of the multitude of selves
- Movement towards authenticity
- Movement beyond basic selfishness toward a focus on being of benefit to the world, and the people in it
- Divine humor and cosmic jokes
- Heart palpitations
- Inspired flows of creativity
- Perception of inner lights
- Bliss, emptiness, ecstatic, and devotional states
- Periods of profound peace and stillness
- Deep depression or existential crises as a result of seeing the world, or the self, as meaningless or insignificant
- Beginning realization of cosmic "I," or inherent potential
- Development of siddhis

When we go beyond the first stage and move into the second, much of the purification fire will no longer be a part of symptomatology. However, the single greatest indicator that we are truly in this stage is the movement away from selfishness. This is a large shift, and is incredibly evident in those who have experienced it. There is really no way to experience any aspect of higher consciousness and not be truly humbled by such an experience.

Some of us who have had a taste of this stage can unfortunately come back to our lives, and our mental limitations can transform such experiences into illusion. Many people want to be led and are more than happy to offer our power up to someone who takes on a label of "guru." With a bit of spiritual power people will be attracted to us and often offer us their power. It can be tempting to see others as lesser for still struggling in large amounts of personal pain and illusion. It takes a lot of willingness to move beyond this and to tell people to look within. We can see throughout history many aware souls who have failed this test, and thus prevented themselves from further realization and evolution.

This is a stage of great responsibility. We move away from the chaotic or "small" self, and understand when personal healing should be attended to.

The physical body is seen as temporary, but essential. Emotions are seen as something to accept and experience, rather than judge or deny. This is the stage of taking great personal responsibility for oneself, and being willing to look directly at what is not working in our lives. In this stage, anger is not something to be resolved but deeply accepted. We do not anesthetize our suffering and we see illusion for what it is: a sign of inner wounding or mental limitations.

In the first stage it is likely that we have seen ourselves as victims, and have healed the times that we have been victimized. We understand self and ancestry, past lives, and other cultural conditionings. We come to terms with what caused someone to victimize or perpetrate harm against others, and we overcome our egoic needs for superiority. We move past being the eternal victims in our lives.

Seeing with clarity how wounded others are, and how locked into illusion and imbalance, can be quite heartbreaking. In this phase we may become quite angry at being responsible when others do not need to, or are not ready to, take responsibility for themselves. There is considerable reconciliation of former selves in this phase, including the realization of how selfish we were prior to this time. There is typically a distancing from the world in order to understand how to traverse it; it is different to see the patterning of others when you have moved beyond much of your own.

What happens in such a world is not perfection as a result of any personal transcendence of limiting material, but of being immersed in a world of pain, of wounding. People may attempt to enroll us in the dramas they have created for us. Learning how to navigate this takes time; it also shows us where we lack compassion and understanding.

We should not expect that people act any better until they have healed and become more conscious. While it is understandable and entirely appropriate to be momentarily angry, or irritated, or simply tired if someone creates chaos in our day, we see this as pointing to what lies unhealed within. In this stage, we see the outer world and the people in it as teachers; it is by noticing our emotional reactivity to people and situations that we can see where our inner divisions lie, and what we still need to heal within.

The path of awakening is not linear. While we are still in human form we will always have personal traumas; the unfolding of consciousness will always reveal what we need to process. However, the vantage point is incredibly different, and we do not get immersed or stuck in such things, or not for very long.

In this phase the awakened flow of consciousness uncoils its second and third coil and kundalini focuses on the solar plexus, heart, throat, and the third eye. The forced flow creates heart palpitations and other symptoms along this pathway. There is still a centralization of the energy within the spine, particularly within the upper chakras, but we are now processing in different areas of the body.

For example, there may be a sense of heaviness in the right lower rib cage with extreme pain and dysfunction, that lasts for weeks, months, years, or just moments. At a certain point this shaking or vibratory energy will move on to the next area to work through, and then extreme pain, dysfunction, and vibratory qualities will happen in that area, as those energies get processed.

We may begin to experience spontaneous vocalizations, speaking in tongues, seeing inner lights and inner deities, and inspired creative flows. We know that we are fully in the second stage when we begin to experience devotional energies frequently, and we are concerned with social and cultural conditioning, rather than personal healing. Also significant is the realization of being of benefit to the world, and the understanding of personal potential in doing so.

The Dark Night of the Soul

We begin to see clearly the karmic connections with friends, family, and others, and will begin to rectify them. This is the stage of the depths of the ocean. We stare into the abyss and confront our atavistic instincts, the secret violence, the aspects of ourselves that want to cause harm and watch things burn. We see our sociopathic aspects, the inner serial killer, the faces of the inner demons that seek to do us harm, our self-hatred, our denial.

We come to terms with our reptilian brain and its basic fears, not through the lens of wounding, but through recognition of our caveman ancestors, our most primal instincts, our inner wildness. In this phase we make large leaps in personal healing as we accept the primitive, subconscious, and most basic instincts/forces within us.

The parts of ourselves that have caused harm—either in this lifetime or others—begin to arise; to face them takes considerable fortitude.

We can also feel deep grief. We find ourselves moving into a type of consciousness that is so unlike what we once were that the former selves need to be grieved. There can be a sense of loss and despair, first because of what pain they were in, secondly because of how little consciousness they had. It is hard to accept, even if we are generally decent human beings, how selfish and greedy and grasping aspects of ourselves are. These are the last bits of ourselves that just want people to like us, just want to go numb, to reach for something, however temporary and illusory, to soothe the pain.

We can also be plagued by a sense of profound meaninglessness. With the loss of the chaotic self that was continually creating drama and distracting itself, a vacuum appears. This is not apathy out of pain or self-protection, this is a profound insight into the noise and chaos of the world, and how we used to participate in it willingly and unconsciously.

We may need to create temporary separation from the world in this phase. We may well know that it no longer makes sense to participate in the drama and meaningless distractions of this world, but we may hunger for them. We may fall into old patterns of behavior that still feel safe or simply fill time. This might bring up a great anger at the world because we are participating in the illusion. Whereas in lesser consciousness states we saw ourselves as separate from the world, above its illusions, in this stage the rage comes from seeing that we help to maintain this illusion because it is safe and known.

Existential crisis is pervasive in this stage. This arises when we see ourselves, as well as others, beyond the personal wounding and we consider the deeper influences and subconscious forces that govern our lives. It is easy to see where others are on their path, and how rare it is for anyone to be beyond the first knot. A true witness state reveals how selfish people are, how most people think only of taking as much as possible from the world, and this makes us angry. However, after healing our remaining selfish aspects we can accept people for who they are with compassion. We can recognize that we need to be a bit selfish while in the human form. We become willing to surrender any thoughts of people changing until they are ready. We begin to work with kundalini, seeing how the resolution of trauma and other issues within the body-mind allows for greater flow. We understand the benefits of conscious participation and of releasing obscuring issues; we see that there needs to be conscious participation for many years to maintain this stage with any permanency.

While we may have periods of ecstasy, bliss, emptiness, and other heightened spiritual states, they are fleeting. Often a profound depression and existential crisis lurks afterwards. This is best expressed by St. John of the Cross, whose *Dark Night of the Soul* describes the crash that comes from experiencing divinity and then falling out of such a state. The phrase has been popularized to mean any type of depression or difficulty on the spiritual path, but those who have experienced higher consciousness states and then found themselves crashing down to earth will understand it in its original meaning.

Even having a glimpse of such states has a deconstructive effect on the personality. In this stage it is not rare to see the illusory nature of the basic "truths" around which we organized our entire reality. We may find it profoundly difficult to accept such perspective shifts. This is especially so because we begin to glimpse our cosmic "I," our true potential, while in everyday reality we may be far from attaining such potential.

Along with a sense of meaninglessness, we may have feelings of self-hatred and not being worthy of receiving grace. This is felt in the heart, and the wounds of the body and the mind begin to be seen through the eyes of the heart. Healing the wounding of the heart is a sacred task. The heart is what carries all of our wounding, the sort of *core wounds* that have created all of the other ones. We may feel existential despair and believe that our previous process, working through the chakra system and all it held, was illusory. However, it was only by working through the chakra system that the core wounds within the heart can be healed.

In the second phase, the experiences of heightened spiritual states become more pure: bliss creates a waterfall of tears, deep ecstasy, the feeling of light and realization of joy filling the heart, a feeling of perfection, freedom, peace—the type of profound settling that feels as if we are sinking into a perfect temperature bath. Moving from those states back into our current consciousness means a feeling of loss of freedom and expansiveness that is nearly unbearable. It is like being in sunlight and then closed up in a dark room.

When we experience higher consciousness due to activation of energetic structures above the head, what we first encounter is typically emptiness. This results in ego death and reorientation, and the initial recognition that we are more than our physical form. This is the Void, still an aspect of our binary existence. In my courses I teach how we can access a light void and a dark void; yin and yang, male and female. Out of those voids emerge the four elements, and then every other bit of differentiated consciousness, including us.

The Cosmic Joke of Becoming Ordinary

States of peace and emptiness can last for moments or even weeks. Beyond this initial state of emptiness or peace is an end to duality. We move into states that are paradoxical and ecstatic, such as the type of dynamic stillness that we see in highly realized souls. We look at them and our first impression is of profound stillness and peace, but looking more deeply we can see a dancing, a lightness, a sense of humor.

There is an ordinary quality to many realized people because they have completed the full circle of this path. They simply attend to their lives, quietly being of service to those around them. There is a cosmic joke in that so many come to the spiritual path to feel special. Notions of being special (and thus separate) through being enlightened or highly realized abound. But awakening allows for us to come home to ourselves, to revel in our ordinary nature, and to heal whatever wounding is within that causes for us to grasp onto the notion of specialness.

If there is consideration of the different samadhi, nirvana, and enlightenment stages described by varying spiritual paths they simply and unfortunately don't line up. Some of them are quite similar, or are using their mythologies and histories to point to the same experience, but I find that they can best be described as qualities: peace, emptiness, bliss, ecstasy, stillness.

In the second stage we see with a clear light, the heart begins to open, and we experience paradoxical states, such as immense tears and profound grief arising in conjunction with ecstasy. Such paradoxical states are the key to self-realization and understanding, and they are found beyond the first states, which consist of singular qualities. Venturing between such paradoxes, or sitting at the conjunction of them, such as between pleasure and pain, or depression and ecstasy, moves us beyond binary experience into spiritual communion.

The heaviness of the first stage lifts, and while there is considerable material here to attend to that is quite dark, an understanding of playfulness develops, and we may develop a rather absurdist sense of humor and the ability to see a sort of "cosmic joke" in many situations. We begin to have insight into our process and false beliefs to the extent that they become deeply humorous. That same gaze looks at the world, and realizes that people are continually showing their deepest wounds to one another by claiming to see it in the other person. We may experience divine states of laughter at our ongoing dramas, at how ridiculous the human body is. We are likely to start to live in a sense of playfulness with the world and ourselves.

Layers of Knowledge

It is at this stage that we really begin to understand that knowledge has layers. We may have understood this intellectually, but the perspective of expanded consciousness pierces through the layers of reality. We begin to understand how something can be true and false at the same time, or true for someone and false for another.

For example, let us take the popular question: "Are spirits real?" For clarity, let's say we are talking about some aspect of the human soul remaining after death that is still a part of the physical or etheric plane.

According to scientific materialist reality they are not real. In another layer of knowledge they are somewhat real. We have a layer in which spirits are real in order to place societal and religious restrictions on people, to make people be good out of fear of going to hell when they die. Then we have layers where spirits are viewed according to archetypes,or aspects of personal psychology. Then spirits are real, but with the distinction that we simply inhabit our space with a wide variety of intelligences and all sorts of spirits and beings, only some of which we are conscious of. This is then true for a bunch of different layers. Then it is not true again, because in a state of oneness neither we nor spirits are particularly real, or are just noise within a web of creation.

Knowledge has gateways, it has thresholds and layers. It is by having this type of perspective that such layers can be seen and known. Before this time the nuance of it will simply not be experienced. We need to pass through those layers to directly experience all of the stages and have direct knowledge of them. People always want to skip to the end; it really is the journey that allows for the evolution of consciousness. Otherwise the nuance is lost, and we need to develop this nuanced perspective, otherwise concepts like *we are all one* become hollow, or even ways for misguided people to abuse their fellow human beings.

Anyone I have met who has experienced this stage develops a deep sense of awe. The feeling of being infinitely small in the vastness that is the cosmic ocean and being held in that flow is indescribably beautiful. It also has the effect of slamming down any last bits of self-importance.

In this stage we move past knowledge. We discover that if we spend enough time following truth (or however we describe our spiritual search) everything sort of falls away. Many of the greatest sages and scholars and poets have come remarkably close to expressing what is indescribable. But the spiritual path needs to be experienced and felt and deeply embodied. Words can only point the way.

One of the least popular things that I can say is that without long-term meditation, this state will not be experienced with any type of permanency. We can benefit from past lives and get there in two years instead of fifty, but it still requires a considerable amount of effort. Most people who assume that they have attained a great state of enlightenment after two years of effort are greatly misguided, and there is an unfortunate trend of people becoming spiritual teachers before they were ever proper students.

To attain a heightened state on a permanent basis, we need a daily meditation practice, keeping the physical form healthy, spiritual practices like self-inquiry and emotional healing. Even if we attain self-realization or anything akin to an enlightened state, to stay in that state we need practices to ensure that the channels of the body are aligned and have flow; we also need to take more and more responsibility for ourselves by looking inward.

The large amount of flow in the body in this stage brings up the most difficult experiences into consciousness where they can flow through like a stream. Automatic static postures and hand gestures lead to heightened spiritual states including ecstasy, rather than processing of trauma. Remaining trauma can simply be witnessed, flow through the system, or be worked on without chaos being created.

We begin to experience full flow on occasion—the meeting and integration of the upward and downward flow and the beginning of the opening of the spiritual heart. However, the difficulty at this stage is that it goes away again. Grace flows downward but that flow only reaches the forehead or the jaw. Meanwhile, kundalini has only unfolded two or two and a half times, so there is still a reserve of potential energy in the sacrum, a strong flow up to mid-back, and then a smaller flow up to the heart and base of the throat. As we feel these types of streams it is very clear in our body where there is flow and where there is not.

In this stage we make large leaps forward in personal healing and personal evolution. Although the previous stage was certainly significant, and needed to be traversed, here we find ourselves in the oceanic depths. During the second phase of kundalini we are willing and able to participate in our own process, however disconcerting, joyful, freeing, and painful it is.

Realization of the Multitude of Selves

There is a certain cosmic joke to the fact that we begin our spiritual journey often wishing to uncover a "true" self—some sort of finally decided, static being. The deep irony is that when we move past our individual wounding, we discover that we are not just one thing: we are a multitude of selves.

We are much more multi-faceted than we give ourselves credit for. Even if we are an introvert we have an extrovert within us. Even if we are peaceful, we have violent aspects. We can love aerobic exercise as well as being lazy and watching television. In earlier stages we see such aspects of self as being at war with one another. If we are a soft person who is attempting to be compassionate, we deny the parts of ourselves that are greedy, grasping, or bloodthirsty.

One of the harshest aspects of this phase is that identities that are submerged at our very depths come forward. It is not pleasant to consider the parts of ourselves that seek to cause harm. It is also not pleasant to be faced with what is still unhealed within us.

However, it is not by denying such things but by truly accepting them that we can understand our complexity. In previous stages this would have created chaos and drama, as these aspects of ourselves are constructed through societal filters that ascribe certain notions of goodness and ethics, and we do not like to think of ourselves outside of such parameters.

Most significantly, we were unable to consider ourselves as anything other than the eternal victim in our own lives. This is the wounded ego, the part of us that is struggling under the weight of being harmed and brutalized, not heard or nurtured. We would project outward anything that we did not wish to heal internally, becoming fascinated by movies about serial killers, fixating in fear on the latest terrorist, decrying others for being filled with hate or for being fake. All the while not recognizing that truly awakening means accepting these aspects within ourselves.

These parts of ourselves are not to be transmuted into societal or personal understandings of "goodness." We must accept even the most vicious, bloodthirsty, apathetic, amoral, and despised aspects of ourselves for what they are, without attempting to change them. That way they can move from being subconscious forces that direct our lives, into a part of our flowing and present consciousness. There is deep power in these aspects of ourselves, and working with these aspects of self through acceptance reveals them to be a source of significant spiritual energy.

Notions of goodness are religious and societal constructs. Compassion does not mean weakness. There can be fierce compassion, warriorship compassion, stoic compassion, angry compassion. It is essential that people who have perspective beyond personal wounding speak out against what is unjust, illusory, and based on imbalanced power in this world.

It is impossible to be singularly good, nor should we be. While we all try our best, we are imperfect creatures and we can create harm. We require a certain amount of selfishness while we are in the human form. We must attend to ourselves, as well as our families and loved ones, first. We can never truly be "selfless" as we must attend to our basic safety, our basic needs, and those of our loved ones.

It is by understanding this that we can accept the aspect of ourselves that must be selfish, that can create harm, that is imperfect, and realize that we simply do the best that we can. If we do harm another, we make amends internally or externally. It is by deeply grounding into our humanity that we can move beyond illusions of a perfected state, and into the type of love for self and others that comes from acceptance of what is.

Addictions and Meaninglessness

The spiritual path gets much harder when we move beyond our basic wounding and get in touch with forces that govern our basic energetic being: creation, destruction, and preservation.

There is a force within us that craves our death. This is not a wounded aspect of ourselves, but a basic force that is propelling us towards our demise. We are born, we live, and we experience death of the physical form. The acceptance of the death impulse within us, the forces that seek our destruction, is necessary during this phase to truly appreciate our basic energetics. This also allows us to move beyond any remaining fears of physical illness and death.

In the first phase of kundalini awakening, addictions and substance abuse proliferate as a result of the purification process and the processing of personal trauma. Yet this can also happen in the second phase, when the initial perspective shift in which we go beyond the ego-mind creates a loss of meaning. Seeing negative forces and atavistic instincts within ourselves is understandably difficult.

In the first phase, our daily reality is struggle enough. Add the emergence of traumatized material coming into consciousness, plus the strangeness of spiritual experiences such as automatic movements and realizations of past lives, and we understand that reaching towards mind-altering substances could stop the process, numb it, or simply allow us to make it through the day.

During the second phase, the perspective has shifted. No longer are we enacting as much trauma in the outer world, creating chaos out of trauma or boredom. A sort of vacuum develops. At the same time we realize with disgust how the world is steeped in ignorance and illusion. This is typically a point at which we seek refuge, distancing ourselves from the world.

There is also a sense of loss here, and a realization of how we previously spent our time. We grieve for our former self and experience a profound feeling of meaninglessness, as well as immense grief at the nature of the world and the people in it.

The only way to move through this phase is by lamenting our former selves and by reconciling the aspects of self that are still selfish and grasping. It is also by opening ourselves up to greater connection: to the earth, to nature, to other people, to the divine, and to greater depths within ourselves. Then we can feel meaningful in our lives again.

It is easy to despair at the state of the world. That despair can flow through us, and we can develop understanding and compassion for people being where they are and the world being what it is. But paradoxically we experience simultaneously a certain level of separation from and a connection to the world on the deepest levels. We are of the world, and deeply connected to it, but we are not in the world in the same way as most people are anymore.

To get through this profound sense of meaninglessness we must realize that we cannot live our lives for only ourselves; doing so does not fill the emptiness within. We are here for our connections, to be of benefit to the world through our unique potential. In actualizing this potential, the despair and feelings of meaninglessness lessen or cease.

Liberation through the Emotions

It is by accepting all aspects of ourselves that we can truly and deeply feel. Many of us are not truly living, but merely surviving. It is by feeling on the deepest levels, accepting what arises, that we awaken. It is by moving beyond the sphere of self that we can begin to witness the pain of others, and the world.

When the size of your bubble increases and you are able to notice more than your own emotional projections, you feel the pain of the world. Exploring what is unhealed within you is always helpful, but in this phase we begin to realize that the world, the people in it, and other beings and intelligences are alive and in pain. There is a collective level of pain in the world that comes from humanity, a wail that comes from the oceanic depths of all those who have suffered. There is a palpable energy of when something traumatic is going to happen on a global scale.

Feeling such things is incredibly difficult. The level of confusion and pain in the world that has nothing to do with us or our personal psychology or wounding is a hard thing to handle for even those with tremendous skill. What is needed for liberation is the ability to feel, to relate, to be in communion, rather than denying, repressing, or controlling the senses or emotions. Witnessing the suffering of another and deeply feeling it within ourselves, allowing ourselves that grief, can free the emotions to flow. Liberation is achieved through acceptance. It is only then that we can realize the skilled usage and inherent power of the emotions. By accepting our emotions, and by authentically experiencing them, we can be liberated through them.

Realization of Identity Separate from Conditioning

Perhaps the single identifying feature of this phase is our awakening to social, religious, and cultural constructs. We are more than just the sum of our wounds, or the wounds that have been passed down to us. It is only by awakening to our personal history, and traversing the first phase of kundalini awakening, that we can understand this.

Prior to this stage, we may feel as if we singularly create the world, or can singularly create our reality. We certainly create a lot of drama for ourselves, and restrict what is possible for ourselves through the beliefs that have emerged from our wounding. But there are societal, cultural, and social constructs in place that very much regulate who we are, and that create imbalances of power in this world. It is only by awakening to these that we can move into realizing that we create this world together.

These constructs form a large part of who we are. Our history, culture, race, gender, and society create specific patterns of relating and being that we are enmeshed with. We can extricate ourselves from such constructs and realize who we are, separate from them. By moving into a witness state with them, we no longer have to blindly carry them out.

Looking towards the parts of us that hate can be incredibly revealing. There is an incredible amount of nuance to this, because at a certain level we are all one. But in this level of reality we are not all the same. By appreciating our differences and seeing the beauty in them, we can move beyond hate and separation both inwardly and outwardly. This may include the realization of how ideologies have been created out of wounding and illusion, and how suffering is perpetuated. But we can still work internally with our reactiveness.

Timelessness and Constructs of Created Reality

We can have a whole host of odd encounters and experiences in this phase. Many pragmatic and balanced individuals often realize when their experiences have moved beyond what is acceptable, even in spiritual communities, and decide to shut up about their experiences.

We can experience processing of parallel selves and other dimensions, full understanding of past lives, or at least many of them, realization of future timelines, and other experiences that are too far from what is considered societally acceptable. Over the years I have learned that it is quite common for people at about the ten-year-mark of daily meditation to begin to have encounters with extraterrestrials. But these people may see the mental-emotional instability of others claiming such experiences and stop discussing their spiritual experiences. In addition, we conflate spiritual experiences in our world with insanity; pragmatic, grounded individuals frequently feel isolated by their experiences, which creates additional trauma.

In this stage we may experience continual states of communion that are felt but cannot be described. Devotion, bowing, feeling of being outside of time and held by something much larger than the self, begin.

Anxiety and fear arise from the deconstruction of the time complex. We have social constructs in regards to when we eat, when we sleep, when we rise, and how we go about our days; when this breaks down we may feel an immense anxiety about adhering to these standards. We can then establish changes in sleep patterns, such as bimodal sleep or less sleep, and in food intake, such as different foods or eating schedule. We live according to our specific needs, rather than through adherence to social construct.

Menstrual Cycle and Kundalini

Although there is rather hazy science when it comes to the understanding of how kundalini impacts the physiology of the body, it is apparent that it profoundly effects the neuro-endocrine systems.

Sexual essence is created in the reproductive organs and is an aspect of creative energy, though such creative energy is typically used in unconscious sexual release or in procreation. We can see how childbirth, ecstatic sex, and other acts of creation engender powerful transformation. They can propel us towards highly conscious states.

Our greatest interface with power or with magic comes at the conjunction of opposites, or in the enacting of the birth-death-creation cycle. Such energies can be used by knowledgeable souls for further evolution of consciousness. Many of my clients have reported difficulties with menstruation due to kundalini awakening. In the first phase, in which kundalini emerges and the first chakra may not be open, the capacity of power and the rising of energy during the menstrual cycle can be a profound catalyst for the kundalini process. Or it may show a woman exactly how much potential is still locked within her system.

If the "snake" of kundalini has uncurled one or two times, a tremendous amount of spiritual power is awakened but still in a holding pattern in the sacrum or first chakra. Women over the years have reported immense pain, as well as ego deaths, as the energy rises through the midline at the start or during the menstrual cycle. They also reported heightened kundalini experiences, as well as bliss or orgasmic states during their menstrual cycle.

Shamanism and Kundalini

There are many similarities between the experiences of some spiritual healers and kundalini awakening. Ideally, spiritual practitioners would have had a kundalini awakening; without the perspective and "sight" that is offered through such experiences, the practitioner would have significantly less capacity to see through their own personal wounding and restrictive ideologies and to view the spiritual realms clearly. Many accounts of shamans tell of feeling lightning pour down, of "fire in the head," and of spiritual power flowing through the system. This power is then utilized to benefit the community, in which the shaman serves as a mediator between the physical world and the natural and spiritual worlds.

The *hollow bone* concept in shamanism is a perfect illustration of how spiritual workers learn to interface with spiritual power. After what is held within is released (the purification process), a clear flow of spiritual power (kundalini) can move through the system. It is then utilized to benefit the community through ceremony and healing. Becoming a hollow bone means that such individuals have the perspective to see the multiple layers of reality as well as ability to interface with power.

There are many different ways to come into spiritual power, and kundalini is one of them. There are all sorts of beings and energies and lineages or currents that are doorways into spiritual experiences; many of them do not require much consciousness or any type of kundalini awakening. There is absolutely no requirement that shamans be enlightened; many are not, and they serve their communities quite well. However, channeling, mediumship and trance states, being "ridden" by spirits, the effects of occult ritual, or other methods do change consciousness quite a bit, either temporarily or permanently, and can lead to kundalini stirring, experiences, or full awakening.

It is not uncommon for magical ritual, shamanism, or energy work to lead to pre-kundalini states, kundalini stirring, or full kundalini awakenings. It is also not uncommon for people to grasp onto the title of "shaman" out of mental-emotional imbalance or the need to be seen as special. However, spiritual work requires the ability to be grounded in this reality as well as many others simultaneously, the stability to be of service to others and to handle difficult or dangerous situations. Becoming a spiritual worker is a lengthy and arduous process. Understanding these aspects of the spiritual path can dispel many of the more commonplace illusions.

Being on a Spiritual Path to Benefit Others

During this phase of kundalini awakening our authenticity rises, along with our clarity and focus on purpose. We gain a clear mind and a sense of peace, as well as the ability to look at the world to see what is unhealed. We have the first realization of the cosmic "I"; through this perspective shift we realize what we uniquely bring to the world. It is by authentically bringing our unique capacities to the world that we can truly understand why we are here and what we are here to do.

In this stage there is a significant switch in core energetics. We move from taking energy in attempts to nurture the system (all energy going in, with very little going out) to bringing what we have realized into the world. We realize that, paradoxically, offering energy and being of service creates more flow through the system and fosters personal evolution.

The spiritual path is now traversed for the benefit of the world, and the people in it. This is a distinct shift, and it is through this shift that we come into states of devotion and bliss.

My Experiences of the Second Stage

It was during this phase that I was able to clearly see and utilize the outer world to see what I still had unresolved inwardly. I noticed patterns of relating, or loops; when the same type of circumstance occurred, I took a hard look inward to see what part of me was creating it or was at the root of it. I began to realize the many karmic links between myself and my clients, friends, and loved ones. This was initially hard to navigate, as the other person had no conscious awareness of such a link.

I began to have immense gratitude for those who were showing me such wounds or where my beliefs were incorrect. A wide variety of different people would come into my life around the same time, all triggering the same unhealed pattern or restricted belief within me. One of these was a certain type of woman who initially puzzled me; up to this point I thought that the spiritual path took direct experience. You did the work, and you saw the results of that effort. But these women had been on a spiritual path for ten, twenty, or even sixty years and they had little or no consciousness. It was because of this type of woman that I stopped offering spiritual guidance appointments to people. She would spend the whole appointment telling me how awake she was, about the fire ceremonies she had attended in Laos, about how she had known someone thirty years ago who was now famous, and about all of the modalities or methods of healing that she had participated in. She would tell me how wonderful she was because she didn't eat meat, or about how she didn't have any anger or shadow anymore because she visited a shaman in Belize.

At the time I held a belief that all it took to become conscious was effort and discipline on the spiritual path. I generally need to feel like I am being of service in my work. I do things wholeheartedly and with passion, or I do not do them at all. These women were not calling me in order to receive a different perspective, or any form of guidance. They were in fact closed to anything I had to say; when I offered any input that varied from their own thoughts they would launch into stories that showed how much they already knew. I began to see and feel compassion for how they had to hold on to such stories because their lives were often a mess, and they still felt empty within.

The compassionate answer is that these individuals may have lacked consciousness, but they had come a long way to even be at the point they were. However, the realization dawned on me that what motivates you on your spiritual path is highly significant. There is a difference between the search for truth, knowledge, communion, peace, divinity, or similar qualities and a spiritual path fueled by self-obsession.

All spiritual paths must start with the self and with self-healing. But that is to get us to the point where we can consider starting to use our spiritual path to benefit others—our families, communities, our ancestry, and the world. If we are only immersed and interested in the self, the bubble around us never expands. We never become more conscious, and never gain the ability to really see anyone around us clearly or apart from our projections onto them.

It was thanks to these women that I corrected a false belief, which allowed for further realization. Over the last five years or so my focus has been on looking to the outer world to see what I have unresolved within. People are forever willing to test me, to see where my boundaries need some work, or to show me where some personal healing needs to take place. This testing has become more and more difficult as I gain more compassion, and sometimes I fail. But such failures always lead to opportunities for growth and inward revelation.

Anyone in this line of work will tell you that mental-emotional instability and the perpetuation of unhealed states is incredibly problematic. The most chaotic individuals that have come my way—those who would no doubt be diagnosed as schizophrenic, delusional, bipolar, or simply disconnected and untethered from collective reality to the point that it is quite painful for them—tend to be therapists or spiritual healers or teachers in my field.

If we are unable to consider anyone other than ourselves, we are self-obsessed, not awakened. Some of these individuals are dangerous; there is no shortage of people in history using spiritual or religious paths to feed delusion, instead of facilitating greater connection. I found myself in this phase in a deep state of concern for such individuals. I often considered quitting teaching as I saw how the field that I was in perpetuated such things, and didn't want to spend my time immersed in chaos with individuals that lacked any type of logic or connection to communal reality.

I began to feel extremely disillusioned about my field of study and started looking at "help wanted" signs at local places of business. I gradually reduced the number of clients that I saw. While I had compassion for how wounded people were, or the sort of spiritual wounding that led to creation of mental or mythic realities, I had little interest in participating in it. I was exhausted by the constant influx of people looking to blame all of their inner problems on spiritual constructs.

Many spiritual movements and teachings are meant to perpetuate illusion. The romanticized and illusory realities are what gain the most popularity in this world, and people reach for them because they give them hope, but they do little to fill the emptiness inside. Few people actually do work of any depth, few are ready to put forth any effort. The modern world perpetuates the idea that spiritual studies are something that can be completed with little or no effort to achieve mastery. All this represents a profound disconnect from the spiritual realms.

Through this I began to realize that my remaining anger and frustration were from a profound grief at being Other. I began to see that I was born into the depths of the ocean (although there are always new depths to be found) and that my struggle was understanding what was going on with myself, and how to navigate it.

My experience of the spiritual realms has always been one of deep connection and sustenance. Even in times of great fear I have recognized the forces of assistance around me. I began to see how much it took for someone to just dip their toes in the water. How they had a choice where I did not. It is so easy to remain in ignorance. It is so easy to remain immersed in illusions of mastery and control and mental imaginings divorced from any type of spiritual reality.

From this point forward I began to have deep respect for anyone who was willing to dip their toes in the water, to wade in. I also let go of any remaining anger or grief I held towards people steeped in illusion. Very few awaken and it is because our illusions are so preferable. They lack nuance, they tell us exactly what we want to hear, they stop us from searching or thinking, and they keep us exactly where and who we are.

Even if our known is a crappy known, we know the parameters of it. We know where our edges lie. To ask anyone to reorganize their reality, especially if they are coming from the shore and dipping their toes in for the first time, is asking a lot. It actually takes considerably more effort than someone like myself who found herself at mid or deep ocean and went from there.

I saw clearly how if we all look in the mirror, we fear our inner madman or madwoman. If we were all to admit how much of a struggle human existence is, how difficult it is being in a physical body with all our trauma and wounding, we would find compassion for one another. We could stop "othering" those who are struggling, or pretending that those struggling will always struggle. We could stop demonizing people who are taking medications or who are making their way through this world the best way that they know how. We all struggle, and it is by seeking support for our struggles that we can make it through.

These individuals allowed me to develop stronger boundaries, to see with clarity that those who are in significant states of delusion or fracturing do not need spiritual work; they need someone who can help them to become functional in their lives again. I began to recognize when people were drowning, when they were too far untethered from reality, and I made peace with the fact that I cannot help everyone.

During this period I also began experiencing flows of inspired creativity. They swept through me, allowing me to get a lot of work done in rather short order. But after the flow stopped, I felt exhausted, as if I had slammed into a brick wall. It took me a while to realize that I could use these flows to nurture myself, to fill myself back up, rather than using all of it for writing or painting.

The most frightening thing for me in this stage was primarily physical. Although I was oddly fascinated by the automatic movements of my hands, arms, and tongue, the throat contractions were more worrisome. I would feel the hyoid (the top of my throat) contract; frequently food would get stuck in the back of my throat. Luckily I was calm enough to know to stand, raise my arms, and swallow until the food would reroute, but the contractions themselves were painful.

During this period I received mouthwork from a CranioSacral therapist to open and realign things; as a result, I was more willing and able to be authentic to the world. I also experienced improvements in my digestive system, and found that a clearer, stronger flow of energy came through me.

Some of the social constructs were difficult for me to traverse, including what I call *socially inappropriate healing*.

During this time I frequently thought of a specific patient of mine. She was beautiful to the point that each time she came into my office, for the first few moments I found myself unable to speak. I have certainly met plenty of attractive people, but this woman was unearthly in her beauty.

When she told me how isolated she was because of her beauty I was unable to consider how deeply this affected her. Later, I kept seeing her face in my mind's eye. I realized that attributes like beauty, intelligence, or physical aptitude can actually create trauma. Due to social constructs, however, we cannot discuss them as we are not supposed to look at them as difficulties.

My experience with this woman helped me see how my intelligence, deep feeling, and perceptual capacities had created a great deal of trauma for me; I was finally willing to look within and acknowledge the pain. I also began seeing on a deeper level how traumatizing many of my spiritual experiences had been, even if they resulted in profound healing shifts. And I recognized the extent of the sacrifices I had made on my spiritual path.

I began to understand my primary motivations for doing things and to look at my addictions. I already knew that I used television to de-stress, but I saw clearly that television energetically shuts down everything around it; I was using it to dull my sensitivity levels. I still do this, but I do it consciously. I accept that I am a work in progress, and do not berate myself when I seek television to provide distraction.

It was during this period that I began to feel grace.

During one of my experiences of feeling grace, I felt a huge wave of energy flow through me, and bolts like lightning entering my crown. I was disoriented, traumatized, and began reliving much of my personal history. I then released a huge layer of ancestral history, and relived my near-death experience. Huge waves of anger rose up and I began shaking. I could not get warm, as I simultaneously felt waves of cold flowing down my body. Two days later I looked in the mirror and saw that large clumps of hair had fallen out of my head where I had felt the lightning hit. I never thought of myself as particularly feminine (this was a pattern that came later to be healed) but having several large round bald patches in my hair was quite upsetting. It was during this experience that a friend, who is an excellent shamanic healer, contacted me and said that she had a dream in which I was hit by lightning.

From that point forward I began experiencing an on-again, off-again flow into my crown that changed my path tremendously. I began to feel devotion, my automatic movements were now of bowing and deep reverence, my arms would go into spontaneous static postures and mudras that pulsed immense amounts of energy through my system. I had a realization of my cosmic "I": what I am here to do, what my full potential is. And I felt that something much larger than myself was inspiring me, assisting me, and flowing through me to help me meet this potential.

If I fully take care of myself during this process—physically, emotionally, and spiritually—I find myself in a wonderful state of flow, high productivity, loving connection to the world. In such states I go into trance, into ecstatic states, into ecstatic posture and dance, and into states of emptiness and then of deep communion. The stillness and dynamism of sitting in communion with nature is perhaps my favorite state, and it is where a great deal of my work is heading. If I go through times when I do not support my process, the flow stops. The ecstatic states stop. But the spiritual experiences do not, and the less effort I put into supporting my own evolution, the more my path feels difficult and disconnected. It is by getting back on the proverbial horse each time I fall off that I find myself back in a state of flow.

This is how I began to realize that we are here to be of benefit, if we can. The purpose of awakening is to "get over oneself" enough to be of benefit to the world. The trajectory of awakening is to be able and willing to offer ourselves to larger and larger constructs and concepts until there is no self left. It is only after giving that we receive back what we are looking for, that we truly fill the spiritual emptiness within.

Healing for the Second Stage

During this stage we are typically interested, as well as psychologically ready, to participate in our own evolution. Daily meditation, physical exercise, and educating ourselves spiritually are all recommended.

Spiritual books are a profound catalyst, if we find the right ones. Without an education, we lack context for experiences. We can easily find ourselves in states that disconnect, or create notions of superiority, simply because we lack the education to understand how much further we can go. If we are open and curious, spiritual education will reveal how little we know, how immense the cosmos is. Humility can develop as we realize how little time we have in the human form.

Flotation Tanks

Sensory deprivation tanks are an incredible resource; they can assist in the evolution of consciousness in ways that are unparalleled. Developed by John Lilly, a neuroscientist on a profound spiritual path himself, the flotation tank is filled with skin-temperature regulated water and Epsom salts so that the body is taken out of the forces of gravity.

While many modern tanks have lights and sound, it is suggested that neither are used, to ensure an isolative, immersive experience. Floating naked without struggling with the forces of gravity, the body adjusts and releases physical pain. This experience has gained popularity with sports figures for the physical release and restoration abilities of a deep rest state, as well as the mental clearing that floating can provide.

Many people today suffer from magnesium deficiencies; as the skin is quite porous and allows for fairly direct access to the bloodstream, Epsom salts can provide a simple way to heighten magnesium levels in the body, reducing pain and providing a relaxation response.

Floating can also lead to changes in consciousness, especially if it is done on a consistent basis. The immersion in water without sensory input can bring heightened spiritual states, as well as spiritual revelation.

Flotation tanks are not suggested for people who are claustrophobic, or who are not looking for additional release or processing. It is not unusual for people to need a few hours after the experience to release large waves of anger and grief, to experience heightened spiritual states or deep fatigue from recalibration of the nervous system.

Bodywork

Bodywork is highly recommended in this phase. It helps us be an active participant in our own process and gives us an outside perspective to ensure that ego dynamics are in check. Working with a skilled professional can help us process substantially larger patterns more readily.

CranioSacral therapy is especially indicated for any phase of kundalini awakening, as it works with the continuum of the spinal cord, skull, and cerebrospinal fluid. Practitioners are often highly educated on the impact of trauma, working with emotions through the physical form, as well as physiological aspects, such as digestive issues, headaches, and other pain issues that can emerge while awakening.

CranioSacral therapy is particularly indicated in this phase because some skilled practitioners work gently with the musculature of the throat both externally and intraorally (inside the mouth). This type of work is called *avenue of expression* work. It is typical for there to be large amounts of trauma and held energy in the area with which we physically and energetically express ourselves to the world.

Without physical and energetic realignment of the structures in the mouth, such as the vomer, the connection between the pillar of energy that flows up our midline to our brain is likely to remain in a state of disconnection. By releasing and realigning the structures of the jaw, head, and mouth, flow can find its way to the brain.

The gentle rearrangement of our physical form through the light touch work that CranioSacral therapy provides allows for nervous system decompression as well as release of substantial blockages. Kundalini awakening will have a profound effect on the physical form, and there are some physical blockages that are so entrenched that it is difficult, if not impossible, to attend to them unless manual therapy (bodywork) is experienced. It is also true that at times our physical structure must change or open to allow for transmutation of mind or spirit.

Kundalini awakening is much more than simply a spiritual or even a mental process, it affects the physical form and has a large physiological impact. We need to work with someone who understands the whole continuum—mind, body, and spirit—instead of its separate parts. Thus we can experience healing as well as significant relief.

In this stage, *Rolfing* or *Structural Integration* is also suggested, especially if we are experiencing significant pain or want deep, physically oriented work to allow for opening of the physical body and greater flow and processing to occur. Work at a deep, structural level can allow for even deeply entrenched and resistant patterns to unearth themselves for further processing emotionally and mentally. Additional individual healing modalities are discussed in a later chapter.

Ecstatic Dance

When we access the primal energies of the body, our deep emotions and inner wildness emerge. These parts of us do not want to tearfully discuss experiences from when we were six years old, or to be suppressed, ignored, shoved into a mental paradigm or turned into love. They want to express themselves, to feel liberated, to release the pent up energy from within.

While other art forms can be pursued, such as painting, singing, playing an instrument, or even listening to music, dancing either by yourself or with others can be quite helpful. A well-led group, for instance Five Rhythms or other ecstatic dancing, can create safety and openness within a field of energy arising from the many participants. Being seen by others while exploring our innate wildness, atavistic instincts, and pure emotion, can move us beyond social conditioning. We see that the deepest and most primal aspects of ourselves can be accepted, and even loved, by both ourselves and others.

These primal aspects link to the base of our power, to deep emotion, and to the most shadowy aspects of self. Trance states, bliss states, and feelings of love can be felt simultaneously with the emerging of our inner wildness. It is only by allowing the deepest aspects of ourselves to emerge that we can evolve into higher consciousness states.

Questions for Self-Enquiry

What parts of me are not authentic?

By questioning what aspects are still wearing a mask, or that do not wish to reveal themselves to the world, we can see what lies unresolved within. Authenticity means embodiment and the release of the false masks we wear. Whereas we can consciously reach for such masks, as one would do to play a role in a film, prior to this point masks show a lack of authenticity and a skewed version of reality. By questioning the aspects of ourselves that are hiding, that do not wish to embody or reveal themselves, or that are pretending enlightenment or superiority, we can see what still feels separated within.

Am I getting lost in phenomena?

It is quite easy in this stage to experience things that the average human being would consider either insane or magnificent, and to hang on to such constructs. We may wish to mentally figure them out, to break them down into something that can be known, and thus controlled.

By asking this question, we realize the fleeting insignificance of much of what comes to pass. We can watch our mind attempt to reduce the ineffable to something that can be controlled, or to relate to it through symbol, myth, or psychological construct.

Most of the higher consciousness states are states of deep feeling, light, or flow. Letting such experiences be what they are, not grasping them, allows us to bring our focus back to what lies unhealed or unprocessed within. We can also understand that our true nature is to permanently abide in them.

Am I fueling self-obsession?

It is easy to use well-meaning constructs, such as "love is all there is," to fuel self-obsession. Such realizations are indeed profound. But they are rarely nuanced enough to meet everyday reality, and we may get lost in flowery or idealized language that does not allow us to meet the world.

What type of love? Is this the soft love that society says is worthwhile, the motherly or fatherly touch the wounded soul craves? There is no way to argue against love, and the experience of deep divine love is a beautiful experience, but such sentiments can perpetuate abuses of power or isolation in a bubble.

You do not need to feel love for someone who has abused you, for someone who is willfully ignorant, who is looking to take as much from the world as they can, or who is seeking to do harm to those they come into contact with. You can understand them, you can see them, you can even love them, but in differentiated reality, that means boundaries. We need to accept and integrate all of our emotions, not just what we call love. One very damaging belief is that we are not "good enough" or "spiritual enough" if we experience any emotion other than love.

Spiritual paths must be nuanced, because such concepts lack depth. What does "love" even mean? How do we enact it in the world? Yes, we can feel love for all that is. We can understand people at rather deep levels. This does not excuse their behavior, even if we can see exactly how they came to be who they are and feel compassion for them.

The victimized aspects of ourselves need to be heard in their pain, their anger, their grief and their fear. They need to realize that those sentiments are not only acceptable but necessary, and feel them deeply—not to be offered a puppy and platitudes about love.

There are stories of cults where concepts such as "divine love" are used to perpetuate sexual abuse or take the power of women and men who are looking for pure sentiments in an impure world.

Moving beyond the knot of the first stage means a shift in the spiritual path: we use the spiritual path to be of benefit to others. This is done by looking within, but even self-reflection can lead to romanticization of spiritual concepts and self-obsession. If this is happening, doing something to be of direct physical benefit to the world, such as volunteering, is indicated.

9

The Third Phase of Kundalini Awakening

In the last phase of kundalini awakening the snake unfolds the last half of its curl, and permanent flow is established from the third eye to the many energy centers above the head. The snake fully unfolding and straightening liberates us from any illusion and aligns us to divinity. If we abide permanently in this state, a deepening of flow and bliss occurs and we drop into divine creative pulsation.

While we can reach this stage temporarily, permanently abiding there gives us the ability to consciously choose our time of death and control our autonomic nervous system (for example, stopping the pulse at will). We understand consciousness creating and witnessing itself.

We fully realize and enact our divine purpose and realize the cosmic "I." The many knots around and within the heart are released, divine power flows through the heart, and immense spiritual power develops.

A clear light flows within, illuminating every cell of the body. We experience the body as vibration. Rather than individual channels, we feel it in the whole physical form, as well as through the energetic field. This is a state beyond knowledge: it is a state of deep feeling and knowing.

Paradoxically, the more we expand, the more we contract in many ways simultaneously. We expand to the point of moving beyond understanding the self as consciousness to a state of witnessing consciousness itself unfold.

This contraction allows for an understanding of how important the physical form is, how short and precious the time in our human bodies, and how dear our connections to friends and loved ones. The significance of sensory experience joins with the ability to deeply feel every single emotion without restriction or illusory beliefs, along with total acceptance of all that is within and without.

Paradoxical states abound in higher consciousness. We cannot process or assimilate them mentally; we can only surrender the need to know everything, or really anything. You may have a spiritual experience that is so profound or so ecstatic that you may not be able to make sense of it for years, if not decades.

I am not convinced that we can abide in the third phase permanently while still in the human physical form. We love to think of the possibility of being perfected, in a state where we are no longer in pain, where we feel safe. We denounce our gurus and teachers for slight imperfections, or even major flaws, and decide that they cannot have higher consciousness.

The realization of substantial spiritual power means that followers and students will naturally be drawn to us. Throughout time people have been attracted to charisma. It has its own magnetism, the sort of illusion and power dynamics that are effective on individuals who are easily swayed by something glittery and false. We need to feel accepted and loved; the wounded parts of us desire to feel special and superior. These wounds are easy to play to, and teachers and gurus have done so for centuries.

The part of us that may have grasped at psychic abilities or powers (the development of *siddhis*) ironically finds itself reoriented towards appreciating embodiment, grounding, and stillness. If there were any type of actual spiritual competition out there, to me it would be who can be of most benefit to the world, who is the most embodied, or who can feel and express the most authentically.

It is also a very paradoxical path in terms of interacting with the world. There is an increased capacity to feel immense compassion and empathy, to meet people and the world for what they are. There is a feeling of continual connection and realization that we are one with humanity. This can result in immense fatigue and a desire to separate from the world and its noise.

If we have any type of awareness and compassion at all, it is heartbreaking to see that society is set up to fail certain individuals, to leave them powerless and unable to get ahead. When we create a bubble around ourselves in which we offer vague platitudes about karma or divine will, fate or the mystery of life, we do not need to contemplate suffering.

Unless we experience them directly, it is difficult to comprehend the ideas that trauma can just mean pain, with little gained from the experience, that often the good people of this world have the most difficulty, and that awareness or higher consciousness brings enormous hardship (but just a different type of hardship than prior).

In more conscious states, the mind is not so easily quieted and placated. Once self-healing occurs to a certain point, the bubble around the self expands, allowing us to see the world more clearly. This is why many of us who have approached the second or third phase of kundalini begin to dedicate our path to others: to friends, to family, to their communities, to the world, and to the divine.

There is so much pain in the world. Letting go of constructs that allow the mind simple anesthetics cease; working with the state of unknowing and uncertainty and fear that creates the need for such paradigms is a necessary part of the path.

The amount of noise within ceases. This is what most people are looking for on the spiritual path: for the wounded parts of ourselves that scream for attention, looping through their wounds again and again, that create chaos, to finally get what they need and quiet down. When we are no longer attending to our wounded children, when we are no longer drowning in the grief of our ancestors, and have deconditioned ourselves from the societal, cultural, and world paradigms, we have the energy and will to shape our reality as we choose.

Societal Conditioning

It is entirely too simplistic to say that we singularly direct the forces of our lives; we are shaped by many things, and many of those things intend to keep us who and where we are. Still, in becoming conscious of these forces, it is easier to gain perspective on them, or even utilize the flaws in them for good.

Societal, religious, and cultural conditioning expects very specific things, and often becomes unappreciative or even violent when implicit or explicit rules are broken. To even think slightly differently in a world with such a limited spectrum of human thought, experience, and ideology, can create willful ignorance or violent opposition from those who rely on accepted conditioning to define and feel in control of their existences.

We are so easily led and told what to believe and be. Our society uses a concept of normalcy that means most people are not living, simply surviving. Many hidden forces influence us. We can sometimes launch into conspiracy theories or aberrations of the mind instead of gaining perspective and liberating ourselves.

In some ways it is true that achieving enlightenment means we radiate divine love to everyone. However, the idea that we can permanently abide in such states has created a great deal of illusion. Some gurus, teachers, and their followers intentionally perpetuate that illusion to create the belief that such an individual is incredibly different. Yet if we read stories about gurus or listen to talks by spiritual teachers over the years, we learn that realized souls get tired, have headaches, feel sick occasionally. They too can go into profound depressions or states of meaninglessness at the nature of the world. Then the spiritual flow returns along with states of heightened consciousness.

Generally I find that kundalini awakens natural aptitudes within us and our unique potential rather than granting any type of genius or sainthood. I was naturally an intelligent person who wrote well and had spiritual aptitude, and so such things were heightened within me and evolved. I have always painted, and although this is a passion of mine, it is not my divine potential, and my capacities have in no way changed. People who have realized their cosmic "I" are math teachers, therapists, artists, actors, engineers, who find that the creative flows that emerge in the second phase allow them to develop their unique capacities and bring that potential fully into the world.

I do not find people with kundalini awakenings to necessarily be better people, or more ethical, at least in terms of societal constructs. It is quite easy to abuse power, to get stuck in ignorance, to believe oneself to be superior. This is especially difficult because people are so hungry for magic, for spirit, for something to fill the emptiness within.

We tend to believe that authenticity or awakening means that we will somehow adhere more to societal and religious constructs of goodness, ethics, or morality. While this may be somewhat true, it does not mean that we adhere to the puritanical ideologies of Christianity and the deeply wounded cultural and societal constructs regarding sexuality.

This often places us at odds with society. Releasing the heavy weight of our wounding—personal, ancestral, karmic—is incredibly liberating, as it is to decondition from societal, cultural, and religious grids; some of the heightened states of bliss, profound love, ecstasy, and dynamic stillness are life-changing. But they place us far outside of what is expected in society. While we may feel compassion for self and other, it is far easier to separate from the world than to be continually immersed in noise and illusion.

Many people are at a point where they just want their thoughts rearranged, to stay within the confines of their bubble of illusion and personal wounding. Many teachers at this point put up strict barriers to ensure that only seekers who are ready and willing to do the work find their way to them. The number of those who are ready to shift, to change, whether it is from having zero consciousness to having a bit, or from being highly conscious to unfolding even further, are far fewer than we imagine.

Most people simply wish for the pain to go away, or create illusion after illusion to not have to face what is unhealed within. Yet we can decide to heal, to evolve, to become. To look straight at the source of suffering within, to see what isn't working in our lives, what isn't authentic within ourselves. Those who decide to will always become more conscious. Those who are looking for something larger than themselves will find it. Those who are disciplined and open and curious and willing to engage humbly with spirit, seeing it as a never-ending vast expanse in which we become smaller and smaller, are those who will evolve the most.

Our bodies and lives will always show us what is out of balance within, and it is by being willing to look within that we can truly transform.

The Spiritual Heart

The end of the spiritual journey is an opening of the spiritual heart. Although the physical heart begins opening prior to this point, the spiritual heart refers to the area around the heart as well as the heart itself. This results in the ability to see and experience the world through the "eyes" of the heart, rather than through the mind.

In Ramana Maharshi's method of self-enquiry, we have a knot two finger breadths to the right of the heart, in the fourth vertebra. This is the *seat of the soul*, and the release of this knot means permanent enlightenment, or a state of clear vibratory flow moving through the whole physical form.

Sufism offers a more complex understanding of the spiritual heart, and considers it a series of five centers. In this system the heart is split into two: the center on the right side means traversing depression, a clouded mind, deconstruction of what remains of the false self. This is a conflict between what is still false in the system versus what is true, and is located by the third rib.

The center of the heart is then connected to the right side via a small meridian; when it is activated there is a flickering between oneness and emotional wounding. Both the right side and the center of the heart open.

The left side of the spiritual heart is associated with the physical heart. When this center opens we experience emotions of love, we hear divine names and music, and we feel devotion.

In energetic anatomy, the spiritual heart is associated with the physical heart, the pericardium, part of the lungs immediately surrounding the heart, as well as the thymus, or the *high heart* which is located a few fingerbreadths above the heart itself.

When the high heart opens kundalini flows through the arms, and divine flow moves through the heart center out into the world. There is a desire to be of service to divinity, along with an increase in overall flow or spiritual power.

We won't understand until this point that deep devotion to being of service in an authentic manner creates immense personal flow—what one gives out one receives back exponentially.

When these centers are opening the flickering can be quite dramatic. Going from profound bliss or peace into a release creating immense depression is hard to manage for even the stablest of souls. At this stage generally it is better to witness what is happening rather than participate in it. We realize how fleeting emotional and other life chaos is, and wait it out.

At times we may feel unworthy to be receiving so much. Grace is an interesting thing. Any parts within that still feel unworthy or inferior will raise their hands. However, our worthiness is in no way for us to determine. All we can do is open ourselves despite feelings of despair that often emerge simultaneously with grace. This allows grace to flow and increase.

The spiritual heart is where we truly contain all of our wounding. We can be authentic, clear, stable, and most of all loving. We can bring so much to the world if we are truly willing to look directly at what is not working in our lives, and to recognize where the wounded aspects of ourselves are seeking to guide our path. We all have a small light within, and that light can grow. We can become more conscious, more aware, more educated, and we can be more compassionate to those around us.

No matter where we are on our spiritual path, it takes dedication, effort, and a willingness to look within. It also takes looking without, and using the world and the people in it to show us what we could still resolve inwardly. It is only by deeply and authentically feeling, by allowing ourselves to move beyond the simplistic and shiny illusions, that we can heal within. We can awaken. We can discover our divine potential and do our small part in making this world better for our presence here.

The cutting of the heart knot creates permanent enlightenment. We see through the spiritual heart, feel divine vibration, and shift into a creation state. This experience is difficult to put into mere words. I will say it is like being held within a cosmic womb, or dropping through the tides and waves of the cosmic ocean to a place in between, to experience a womb-like divine creative pulsation. We witness consciousness itself—expansion and contraction; emptiness and fullness; void and non-void.

My Experiences of the Third Phase

I have experienced this phase only three times; each time it was quite brief. My reality completely shifted to the extent that I emerged from each experience in existential crisis and in the profound darkness of depression.

I am doubtful that this shift can totally be sustained within the human form. There are many words that could attempt to describe such a state: expansive pulsation, embryonic, dynamic stillness. A witness to creation creating itself.

The first time I experienced this state I was still in the first phase of my awakening. I was watching the news on television and saw a photograph of a woman with tears streaming down her face as she realized that her child had been shot. It showed her agony, her utter defeat as her worst fears became a reality. I felt tears well up in me as I witnessed something so profound, but then I stopped myself. In a world like ours, we are not supposed to cry, to feel, or even to empathize. Then I realized what I was doing and let myself cry, witnessing this woman's pain.

I suddenly felt something so large, so expansive, and with such flow that I could not fathom it. The back of my head shoved back to my shoulders, exposing my throat, the rush of energy through me so expansive that I found myself in ecstasy. But then I went even beyond that, and witnessed myself in ecstasy as cosmic consciousness flowed through my body.

I found myself deeply bowing and expressing profound gratitude, tears streaming down my face. I felt unworthy, I felt unloved and small, and understood through this first experience how much pain we experience as humans, what struggle we go through, and how short life is.

I saw how insignificant humanity was, how meaningless in the grand scheme of things. This was entirely paradoxical and experienced as I was simultaneously grieving with this woman who had lost her son; her pain was so profound, her loss so significant, her story needing to be told.

This completely reordered my reality. Many of the things that I was so anchored into were an aspect of me attributing such significance to humanity. Moving away from this created huge rifts in my identity and my daily life. At the same time it freed me to authentically feel, or to authentically show my feelings outwardly, without any type of mask, for perhaps the first time in my life.

This reorientation took an incredible amount of time. I cannot claim to have totally integrated the experience, even eight years later. I realized that how I was looking at things was incredibly small.

I sobbed for hours, a sort of cathartic release in which I reoriented to feeling deep gratitude for my experiences. Prior to this point, I was angry at my sensitivities; I held an incredible amount of animosity towards those who could simply wade in the ocean while I felt myself plunged into its depths. Others did not wake up some mornings to hear the earth screaming. They didn't need to feel the wail of the ocean and all who have been lost in it. They didn't know how difficult the spiritual awakening process actually is, and how much suffering and personal fortitude it takes. They didn't need to take personal responsibility for themselves, to be Sisyphus constantly and continually rolling that boulder up the hill.

This was the first time that I saw lights within, the forms of deities and eyes in my chakras, the opening of my spiritual heart. I realized that my efforts were leading me to a specific place, and I had an eagle-eye view of how I had been led to it. I heard a small voice within telling me that it was time to let go of the rest of the pain of being at such oceanic depths, and of the pain of others who were unable to access or meet me at those depths.

Awareness is not always a gift, and consciousness brings unique hardships. The part of ourselves that is so wounded and noisy and brings chaos does clear away. We can individuate from the conditioning of the world, we no longer blindly react or project or loop. Or we are conscious of when we do loop, and simply heal whatever wounding is behind it. And there is still pain. There is the pain of the human physical form, gradually moving towards the death process. There is the pain of awareness, of being someone who has a different perspective, what it means, and what to do with it. Being aware of more than our own selfishness and seeing others means a recognition of their pain and what they carry. Truly witnessing from this perspective is quite lonely, even if paradoxically we feel incredibly connected at the same time.

It was from this perspective shift that I realized that my life should be one of spiritual service. I recognized that the part of me feeling Other was immersed in wounding, and the selfishness that arose from it. I was still very immersed in the self, but something small began emerging within me—the seed of realizing that my purpose here was to be of benefit to others. My path and personal hardships were not in vain, or not a force that was acting against me. In being authentic, in being of service through realizing my cosmic "I," my otherness could bring benefit to the world, if I was willing to step away from the pain of being Other.

My practice became more focused on spiritual work, specifically writing and teaching. It was very difficult for me to give up degrees and certifications and all of the things that took me so much time (and so much money). Four years of graduate school and the endless workshops and achievements that I had attained were merely preparatory work for what was emerging within me. I had needed to have context and education for a process like this to unfold. I experienced immense gratitude towards the part of me that was so confused and lost, so frenzied and bent on proving herself.

The decade that it took for me to personally heal, to fully focus on my path at the exclusion of all else in my life, was not something to lament. It was not something to use to create distance between myself and others who could never understand such a path. It was something that was necessary, and something that had evolved me beyond so much pain and confusion.

My experience in 2016 of "dropping through" occurred during meditation. At this point I had meditated for almost twenty years, and due to my early Zen Buddhist training I tended to disregard a lot of the imagery that came up. It was not that such things were not relevant, but I am grateful for this early path as it allowed me to not get stuck in any phenomena, not even bliss or profound states of peace.

Yet this was initially at odds with a lot of my shamanic training, which works with symbols and spirits and the senses in a way that Zen would disregard, or see as byproducts on the path. But pairing the two together has allowed me to experience things fully and dynamically, as well as to avoid attaching mental significance to things. Generally I find that if a message or something else needs to arise, it will do so, and I do not need to sit for hours or decades figuring it out. If we don't let go of this need to know at a certain point, we can drive ourselves a bit crazy trying to figure out what has happened. This teaches deeper surrender.

In this experience I began to feel my whole body as vibration, each molecule separating; a feeling of flow came over me. I felt myself as part of the large ocean of cosmic consciousness, and saw myself dropping through this into something that was womb-like—pulsating, still, and yet dancing at the same time. In my biodynamic CranioSacral therapy training we had talked about dynamic stillness, but this was the first time that I truly knew in an embodied way what that meant.

My heart opened quite painfully, and I realized in an instant how selfish I still was. It was in this moment that I realized how precious the human body is, how important embodiment is, how important our human connections are in the physical form. How our senses are meant to be open, to be authentic, to be in free flow.

I felt lights fill up my head and flow through my heart, and experienced music that filled my senses. What emerged for me was a profound realization that my path has very much to do with authenticity. I am actually a fairly private person, and for a long time I stopped myself from writing this book. There was an immense struggle between the aspects of myself that wished to remain private—that wanted to move to a cave or someplace far from humanity so I was not so immersed in the noisy chaos of the world, to separate myself from the projections of students and clients—and the parts of me that wanted to describe this process authentically because it is direly needed in this world. I felt the urge to look within to see where my resistance was to writing about this period of my life, and did healing work to move beyond that resistance.

I still jokingly say that my idea of an ideal vacation is that to be dropped from a small plane into a cabin for a week with nobody else around for a thousand miles. Ideally that cabin would have modern plumbing, WiFi, snacks, and Netflix, and would be located on land that had never had a massacre on it.

I do have full recognition at this point that it must be difficult, if not impossible, to be enlightened in the modern world. I recognize that people wish to believe themselves to be all sorts of things, but in general I notice that people who have experienced states like this have a tendency to drop out of the public sphere.

Spending a decade at the exclusion of all else to understand my spiritual experiences, my perceptual or psychic capacities, and my awakening process, was of course for myself, but hopefully will allow others to move through their process, dispel illusion, and move beyond the vapid romanticization of the spiritual path. Now being five years past that decade my path has been paradoxically quite a bit easier as well as immensely more difficult, and gratifying in many ways. But offering myself of service in this way is very much at odds with my desire to be left in solitude; I sometimes wonder how writers like JD Salinger and HP Lovecraft, who were too far outside the norm to be able to navigate humanity, would fare today in the era of social media.

My life became more and more devotional. I experienced huge waves of creativity flowing through me. My automatic movements became static, bowing, in deep reverence. Ecstatic states including ecstatic dance came several times a week, as long as I stayed consistent with my daily yoga, meditation and spiritual practices, and ate well.

The last experience of this state of witnessing consciousness came on the tail end of an ecstatic state. Again I felt an opening of the area around my heart, as well as a feeling of my whole brain filling up with light. This ecstasy came oddly as a result of successfully hanging a few pictures. I am in no way mechanically, mathematically, or otherwise inclined, so successfully using a level to hang several pictures evenly was quite a feat for me. But looking at my work being correctly done immediately began putting me into a trance state of bliss. Then I moved past that state.

I felt that same pulsation, that feeling of being in the womb, of profound stillness and peace, and simultaneously huge flows of energy. It felt as if I was in this state for hours, but only a moment or two had passed. I wish I could describe more clearly what happened or emerged in those moments, but words fail me.

What I can say is that each time I have had such an experience my life has profoundly changed. I feel more, I realize more and more what I am here to do. I recognize who I am.

I feel such flow within me sometimes that it is hard to contain; I can ride the flow for hours, emerging exhausted afterwards. Such things are still hard for me to calibrate or make sense of. I know that I am doing the work that I am meant to be doing, and that my job is to be as authentic as I can, while understanding that with each new perspective, that authenticity may change. Each experience has allowed me to be more compassionate towards myself as well as others.

Each experience has also displaced me, even if paradoxically I feel so much connection. I realized after my second experience in 2016 that focusing on what is disconnected within me is where the greatest advances in healing occur. Connection to ourselves, to one another, to nature, to the world, to the divine, to all that is—we are meant to be in a state of flow, a state of connection, and it is by seeing where we are disconnected that we can heal.

These types of experiences have returned me full circle, so to speak. I used to get such pleasure from being in simple and direct communion with the natural world. Sitting by the birch trees with the cold Minnesota sun when I was a child, I felt what the world and each being, each leaf, and everything around me had to say through simple silence and reverence.

I am incredibly grateful for my spiritual path now. My experience of devotion and direct revelation only increases, despite the difficulties and pains of awareness and of navigating a world that is so immersed in selfishness. I know now that the work I am doing is the work that I am intended to do. My cosmic "I" is emerging, sometimes only briefly, and sometimes with such clarity that it destroys any illusions that remain.

Each experience of such vastness has allowed me to see clearly where I am on my path. I am willing to evolve with my consciousness, to be a participant in the process, and to see clearly what remains within me that is still locked in illusion.

This world is so beautiful, and has such pain. It is by allowing ourselves to become who we are intended to be, and by witnessing both the beauty and the pain, that we can awaken.

10

Diet, Lifestyle, and Kundalini

Diet and lifestyle choices can make all of the difference with a kundalini awakening. Our choices of food create fuel in many ways for our system; while most of us are well aware of this on a physical level, on an energetic level we may not be aware of the full extent of its importance.

When we digest, we not only digest to provide physical nourishment for our physical bodies, but we also process our emotions, daily experiences, thoughts, and actions through the same system. If we provide proper nourishment and attention to what our individual bodies need, we have a much smoother experience of kundalini awakening with fewer symptoms or difficulties. In this way we assist our own awakening and provide the nourishment that our body needs to turn differentiated or unrefined energy in the body into refined energy.

If we are poorly nourishing our bodies, not listening to what they need on an individual basis, we will not have enough fuel for the unrefined energies of the body to refine themselves and feed this continuum, allowing for expanded consciousness and a full flow of energy into the brain through the sushumna.

Even if we are well meaning, we may ascribe to heavily restricted ideologies about what foods to eat. While specific diets can provide a model for us to follow, especially if we lack education in nutrition, it is all too easy to use diet to perpetuate mentally restrictive paradigms.

We may aspire to "do no harm" by our choices of what to eat and where to shop. We could have the best diet in the world but if our actions and thoughts do not include compassion for others and an awakened understanding that the world does need to act according to our particular ideologies, or if we believe that we are superior to others due to our dietary choices, we may in fact be doing immense harm. We may be harming ourselves through our sense of separation, and harming other humans by disregarding them and lacking in compassion, or by believing they should follow our own mental paradigms and dietary ideologies.

The other fuel for the kundalini process is our thoughts and actions. It is by seeing where our inner and outer divisions are, recognizing that people are where they are, that we can use diet as well as our thoughts/actions to become more conscious. We can become more accepting and loving towards ourselves and others, and move beyond our need for people to act in accordance to our values. From a place of compassion we can educate those ready to hear, rather than from a place of hatred, wounding, egoic superiority, or imposing our personal ideology.

Awakening is the transcendence of ideology—even helpful ideology. What food we eat when going through any spiritual awakening, including a kundalini awakening, has nothing to do with ideology or food trends. It is about a felt sense, an embodiment. Through connection with the physical body and our intuitive capacities we realize that the body will tell us exactly what it needs during this process.

Traditional Ayurveda, Chinese medicine, Tibetan medicine, and many holistic or Eastern nutrition programs advocate the consumption of meat. Such systems look at the individual and our unique makeup, what climate we live in, what season it is, and what brings us into balance again, rather than a "one size fits all" model.

In the West, our diets include heavy meat, "non-foods" that have heavy chemicals and hormones added, and a lack of vegetables and nourishing foods. Such a diet has perpetuated disconnection from our bodies, and makes us reach for sugars, starches, and carbohydrates as fuel sources. We are over caffeinated, eat too much meat, lack nutritional education about how to care for our bodies in a healthy way. Our lifestyles cause us to reach for what is fast and easy, rather than what would properly fuel our bodies.

Due to the huge transformations going on in our bodies during kundalini awakening, we may go through periods when we are unable to eat meat, or anything much beyond rice. Meat is energetically heavy, and physically difficult to process, but if we are experiencing an awakening this is not a question of ideology; we may have issues with the texture of meat, feel grief or fear after eating meat, or be unable to digest it. This may last for weeks or it may be a life-long change. It is by checking in with the body, developing a relationship with it, that our unique needs can be understood.

It is typical for those experiencing awakenings to include more vegetables in the diet overall, and to go through periods of vegetarianism or even veganism. This could be a permanent change. However, even the best dietary beliefs can be transcended for further awakening. We may not change our diet, but we will stop from getting hooked into a mentally-based ideology or a superiority complex. We can move into greater spiritual considerations and liberation from even the most compassionate of beliefs.

After we have processed our wounding regarding food issues—whether from this life, a past life, or ancestors and others who may have starved—we can form a personal relationship with food again. The body begins craving what it needs to stay in balance; at the very least, it clearly tells us what foods cannot be processed.

Well-cooked vegetables, rice, and congees can serve the body well during the most tumultuous of times. In my own process, I went through a year-long period where I was only able to eat rice, and another six- to eight-month period where I was on a diet that consisted mainly of rice and avocados. This was not a balanced diet, but anything else would make me quite ill. This is not unusual for people who are truly undergoing kundalini awakenings, especially for those who have previously not tended to diet well.

My diet prior to this had large amounts of sugar, soda, carbohydrates, processed meats, spicy foods. I ate when I was supposed to eat, and in rather large amounts. It was part of my upbringing to finish my plate, and Western society has enormous portions. Our brains do not kick-in the satiated response unless we take breaks during our meals, and we often distract ourselves during mealtimes so we do not process fully that we are eating. This results in not understanding that we are full until we are overfull, or in reaching for foods to provide emotional nurturing to fill the sense of emptiness within.

Through an elimination diet as well as personal exploration I found that my previous diet had resulted in my system being unable to process gluten, spicy foods, and nightshades. I also drastically reduced the amount of dairy and meat in my diet. Eating small meals throughout the day rather than large meals helped quite a bit, while healing the societal impulse to eat at specific times of day freed me (except when eating socially, of course) to eat when I was actually hungry. By eating this way I began to hear clear messages about what foods to eat and when.

I find that those undergoing kundalini awakening naturally go through periods when they do not eat very much, or fast, or their requirements for food intake will be lessened temporarily or permanently.

Overall, the systems of Chinese medicine and Ayurveda have the most to offer nutritionally. This includes advice to eat with the seasons, individualized guidance regarding what would work best for our individual constitution, and an understanding of the importance of all the flavors and colors. In the modern world we have a reliance on sweet and heavy foods, and do not explore the full range of tastes that would allow for the best health: sweet, sour, salty, pungent, bitter, and astringent. We especially lack bitter and astringent foods; all tastes have different synergistic effects on the body; we need all tastes to be a part of our diet.

Eating with the seasons and a deep understanding of the energetic impact of foods has been a part of Chinese medicine for centuries; many practitioners are also versed in *functional medicine* as well as Westernized nutrition. If we lack knowledge of dietary needs or suffer from a great deal of digestive dysfunction, a highly qualified practitioner of Ayurvedic or Chinese medicine can recommend a diet specifically tailored for our individual constitution, bringing it into balance using the full rainbow of colors and tastes.

Those experiencing kundalini awakenings do seem to do quite a bit better with constant, small quantities of food. What this food is depends on where we are in the process. Due to the trauma that can occur from to the rerouting of the digestive fire, which can lead to sickness such as nausea, vomiting or diarrhea, we may hesitate to switch diets, or add on foods, even if our body is craving something new. This is especially true if we find ourselves emerging out of a period when we were unable to eat anything except for small amounts or an extremely limited diet.

It is important to heal the trauma that can occur as a result of spiritual awakening and to process the fear that results from experiencing significant digestive distress. It may be necessary to find a bodyworker, such as a CranioSacral therapist, who can work with the abdominal organs as well as the enteric and nervous system to release body-held or physiological shock. By listening to the body, we may realize that we are beginning to crave things that seem out of the ordinary, such as butter, fats, cheese, or meats, and introducing those elements back to the body slowly.

Overall, the digestive system more readily absorbs simple foods, for instance, recipes that do not have a large number of ingredients, and food that is well cooked. Plant-based diets, or diets that include a lot of vegetables and less meat, typically work best for most people, kundalini awakening or not. Raw diets composed of plants and fruits work well for yogis and others who have a stabilized system. If we live in a cold climate, and have an aged or significantly distressed digestive tract from years of neglect, cold and raw foods will lead to intense distress instead of healing. It is always necessary to see where we are individually in terms of our health, our local climate, or the season, and what our own body needs to come into a state of balance. Then we can provide it with the fuel for further awakening.

Diets and Fasting

Eating Locally

Some herbalists, nutritionists and chefs espouse the idea that herbs and foods that come from the area where we live provide the greatest benefit. This often ensures that we eat with the seasons and the cycles of the earth. We are energetically intended to cycle our energies with the earth, as well as the lands that we live on. Food and herbal products that come from these lands would then energetically be a greater match for our systems; they may also be produced by people who have more conscious awareness and a deeper relationship with what they are growing.

Head-to-tail, or using all parts of an animal, is a modern trend that has long been practiced by those who live in wilderness and must forage for food for their families. Those who are in an intimate relationship with the earth and who hunt or have farms are often highly conscious when it comes to preservation, and are interconnected to the land and to the animals they hunt, in a way that even those with the best of intentions but are disconnected from the earth and their food choices are not.

Herbs, mushrooms and other locally sourced vegetables and fruit have an energetic vitality as well as a similar energetic structure to our own, as we are living and experiencing the elements, the cycle of seasons, and other factors together.

While eating locally and with the seasons is helpful, the cost may be a prohibitive factor for some, depending on the area. There is also a genetic factor here; for example, someone originally from Jamaica may eat a variety of spicy foods, as well as fresh, cold fruits, intended respectively to promote sweating and circulation, or to cool down the system. If that person now lives in Chicago (which is quite cold and often damp) there will still constitutionally be a craving for such foods, even if the local climate would require a different type of diet altogether. The task then is coming into balance between the two worlds.

Fasting

There are many benefits to fasting; giving the digestive system a chance to rest and rejuvenate has been shown to be helpful on many levels for those who have significant digestive issues, or who are interested in practices of longevity or aging well. This is also true if we want our system to spend time on more spiritual or energetic concerns, rather than the processing of physical food through the digestive tract.

Fasting once a week, or when called to do so, can allow healthy individuals to immerse themselves in meditative or spiritual practices with increased energy and clarity. There are many spiritual rituals that involve fasting to create a change or shift in consciousness, or to purify the system so we can communicate more easily or exchange spiritual energies. Many of us experiencing awakenings, including kundalini awakenings, may notice that our bodies naturally do not want food during certain days or during certain phases of our awakening.

However, fasting can create imbalance and difficulty for those who are in ill health, have considerable physical issues, especially having to do with blood sugar, or those who have not worked through the emotional layers of eating or of being deprived of food. What can be better for someone if the body is significantly out of alignment is a small meal or small amounts throughout the day; better still is working with a practitioner who focuses on diet.

Mono Diet

A mono diet, or eating small amounts of a single food at a time, is helpful if significant digestive distress is experienced. Simple, well cooked foods, such as a single vegetable with a dash of salt or a bit of butter (or ghee, or healthy oil) is typically well absorbed by the system. Overall, simpler preparations involving fewer ingredients are beneficial when going through spiritual awakening.

However, it is essential that enough calories and nutrition are taken in, especially if this method is used for periods of time. While eating six to eight times a day (or even more) may sound inconvenient, the continual influx of small amounts of simple foods can be life-saving if we feel as if our body is rejecting everything we take in.

If using this method, larger batches of simple foods can be made and refrigerated or frozen for later usage. Some baby foods that have high nutritional value can be substituted if there are periods in which the body is unable to take in solid foods, or if energy levels dip to the extent that cooking is not a possibility.

Paleo Diet

The paleo diet consists of grass-fed meats, healthy oils, fresh vegetables and fruits, eggs, nuts, and seeds, and avoids dairy and grains. It comes from the idea of eating what our ancestors who hunted and foraged ate. While this can be a helpful model to nudge us in the right direction, we do not really have a clear understanding of what our caveman ancestors ate; we are not biologically identical to our predecessors, nor are the foods that we eat. We have selectively bred and evolved, as have our foods. Taking one small segment of our genetic history and pinning it up as an ideal doesn't make much sense. What makes sense is returning to whole foods, real foods that provide large doses of nourishment for the physical body.

What could be eaten or foraged by our genetic predecessors varies wildly from one region to the next, and so the idea of a monolithic sort of "caveman" identity is inaccurate, as is not understanding that modern evolution and ingenuity has its place dietarily.

This diet can also become highly restrictive to the point that many people lack the financial resources or willpower to follow it. However, it is incredibly successful at cutting out processed foods and refined sugars, and making us highly conscious of what we are taking in our bodies. It also has many communities and like-minded individuals that can offer emotional and practical support. While the origins or ideologies of such a diet may not be terribly sound, it can make a tremendous impact, especially if this is the type of diet that your body craves or you are looking to make a large shift in your dietary habits.

Fermented Foods

We can remedy the lack of bitter and pungent foods, as well as the earthen sort of taste called *umami,* by introducing fermented foods into the diet. While kimchi is the most popular, there are many different types of fermented foods available, such as yogurts and sauerkraut.

Fermented foods can provide a rich source of vitamins, the tastes absent from the Westernized diet to rebalance the system, as well as a natural source of probiotics, which introduce helpful and necessary bacteria to the digestive tract.

It is typical for most Westerners to at first dislike fermented foods; this is because we are unused to the taste and need to build up an understanding of how beneficial such foods are for the digestive tract. Introducing fermented foods slowly can allow us to acquire the taste for such foods, and even to crave them, as our system makes the link between becoming healthier and fermented foods.

Food Elimination Diet

If there is significant digestive distress or allergic response to foods without understanding the source (such as itching, rashes, difficulty breathing, heart rate increases, or feeling ill anywhere between thirty minutes to six hours after eating) a food elimination diet is recommended.

A typical food elimination diet removes gluten, dairy, soy, eggs, corn, pork, beef, chicken, beans/lentils, coffee, citrus fruits, nuts, and nightshade vegetables from the diet for a period of at least one month. If there is significant distress, two months is really suggested. There are various ways to do an elimination diet, but removing all of the commonly irritating foods at once to give the digestive system the time to heal and release held irritations is really necessary to get the best information.

It is always a struggle to convince people to change their diets, even for a short period of time, especially to such a restrictive diet. What we eat influences everything from how we are doing emotionally to our mental capacities; it can even create massive pain, such as the impact of arthritis and other systemic inflammations. Many people walk around feeling horrible not understanding that their diet is a large reason why.

After the month or two of the elimination diet, one food is then reintroduced for a week or two to see if there is an allergic response. Typically this response will be quite clear, including headaches, rashes, difficulty breathing, and other pain issues. It is common during the elimination phase to ask "what in the heck can I eat?" The answer is rice, many vegetables, and fish, turkey, and lamb as well as healthy fats.

Food allergy testing can be quite expensive and unreliable, because if your system is inflamed, it will show an allergic response to pretty much every food. While the elimination process seems like a huge issue for most

162

people, those who are experiencing significant pain or digestive distress will find their efforts worthwhile. The information garnered from a reasonably short period (typically two to three months) shows us which foods create health and which create havoc, leading to a much healthier life.

It really is best to find a practitioner who can guide you through this process, such as a holistic nutritionist or a Chinese medicine or Ayurvedic practitioner specializing in digestive disorders. But there is also a wide array of information online that can help you understand the process.

Congee

Congee, a type of rice porridge, is a staple of many Chinese households, although varying forms can be found throughout Asia and Africa. It is particularly used in Chinese medicine to help those with fatigue, who have poor digestive systems, who are going through difficult emotional times, or who are experiencing significant imbalances, such as cancer and cancer treatment.

Rice is boiled until it becomes a porridge-type consistency. There are many different ways as well as ingredients that can be utilized to make congee (also known as *jook*) and a "lazy way" of creating a congee is to use day-old rice from the previous night's meal and add some chicken broth and other ingredients to create breakfast.

In times of immense hardship, lamb or other slowly cooked meats can boost the energetic reserves of the body. Just as with the American favorite, chicken noodle soup, we can feel a sort of warmth and soul-level emotional support from quite a simple meal. During times of particular digestive distress, congee is something that will be accepted by even the most hesitant and tumultuous of digestive tracts.

Congees are a perfect vehicle for any type of vegetable and meat, but a congee made with rice in chicken stock (or with chicken bones and chicken stock), ginger, soy sauce, and scallions is a simple way to create an easily digested, nourishing meal. Extra can be made and will keep for about two days.

To make congee, add rice to cooking liquid (such as stock), as well as any bones (optional). Cook, letting it come to a boil and then putting it to simmer, gently stirring on occasion, until it has a creamy consistency. This takes approximately 60 minutes. Then add any other ingredients and cook an additional 30 minutes (the recipe takes about 90 minutes of cooking time overall). If raw meat is added, that would go in at the beginning, as can ingredients like ginger to bring flavor. The more that you stir the better the consistency gets, and the less it is likely for rice to stick to the bottom of the pan.

Vegetarian or vegan versions, as well as shortened time versions utilizing a rice cooker, are quite easy to find and allow for a similar experience of an easily digested, hearty, and nurturing food.

Meditation Advice

If the kundalini awakening process is overwhelming, consider ceasing all spiritual activities, including meditation. This is the typical advice for anyone drowning in the process, especially during the first phase, when it is typical for us to be unable to read, meditate, or want to create more spiritual experiences for ourselves. If kundalini emerges in an unprepared system, spiritual activities and seeking can be like adding gasoline to a wildfire.

For those who are not drowning in their process, it is essential to have a daily practice of meditation. Our minds are quite noisy. Meditation gives us tools to regulate, quiet, and work with our mind, leading to a practice of self-inquiry. What has become popularized in Westernized society is basic mindfulness and present moment awareness; while this is helpful and a part of meditation, it is not the totality of what meditation has to offer.

In the first phase of kundalini awakening, it is best to find a progressive relaxation meditation. This is also where I suggest those who have never meditated before begin. This can help to support the nervous system, encourage sleep, and release physical tensions and held emotions.

The practice of mantras engages the mind and gives it a point of focus. Immersive silence is difficult for those just beginning to practice meditation; mantras and progressive relaxation give the mind something to "do." Later, other meditative paths, such as silence and witnessing, can be explored.

A self-inquiry practice involves deeply questioning within and looking towards what isn't working in our lives. We can awaken by utilizing the outer world as a resource for what is unhealed within. *The Body Deva* describes such a method of self-inquiry; another one is the simple questioning of Ramana Maharshi's self-enquiry.

Yogic breath, or practices that utilize breath as a vehicle of consciousness, are another aspect of meditative practice that can allow for differentiated qi and/or kundalini to flow through the body. Learning about the many different ways to regulate and work with breath, from gentle to cathartic, produces deeper understanding and transformation of the system than breathwork that singularly focuses on catharsis.

If there is an imbalance related to pingala or ida, alternate nostril breathing can allow for balance to return to the system. For example, if pingala is overactivated, bring the breath in through the left nostril (ida/lunar), visualize coolness, and then breathe out fire through the right nostril (pingala/solar). Breath brought into the sushumna can provide further awakening, but breathing towards this channel can create uncomfortable activation for those experiencing difficulties with kundalini awakening.

There are a lot of quite lovely Buddhist practices, but I find that Zen Buddhism has a lot to offer to those on any type of spiritual path. Looking at any experience or even siddhis (psychic powers or abilities) as a byproduct of the process can keep us from getting wrapped up in our experiences, which can be a common barrier to further progression.

Finding a proper teacher or practitioner is discussed in chapter 12, "Finding Assistance." It is unfortunate that spiritual study is no longer considered an in-depth field taking many decades to master; it is all too easy to find teachers and practitioners who announce mastery and competence with little or no training. That said, there are many lovely teachers who provide programs of spiritual practices; see what works best for you. Gaining a foundation in meditation, and turning it into a daily practice, ideally with a competent and clear teacher, is incredibly helpful in the process of kundalini awakening.

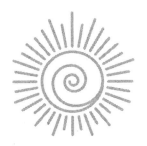

11

Herbal Supplements
and Herbal Support

A huge range of supplements and herbal products can be of assistance during the kundalini awakening process. It is ideal to find a competent herbalist or other practitioner to show you the way, or to find herbs specifically geared towards your system. However, with a bit of education, self-administration of herbs or herbal supplements can be of immense benefit.

The information below is in no way intended to be comprehensive; rather it is a sampling of common products that have been found to be of assistance during the kundalini awakening process.

For those experiencing kundalini awakenings I recommend that you start out simply with one herb or product for a few weeks: this ensures that you understand the reaction to that herb as well as its efficacy. Simpler herbs and products, as well as liquid formations, are more easily digested, and thus better for a system that is dealing with overwhelm.

Most store-bought products will have a suggested dosage. If you are particularly sensitive it is suggested that you start with a third or half of the dose for at least a few days and then build up the dosage as necessary. It is typical for those undergoing spiritual awakenings overall to need less in terms of dosage to receive therapeutic benefit. However, if there is no noticeable change or shift within two or three weeks of regular usage, either increase the dosage or consider a new herb that you can take instead of or in conjunction with the herb you're already taking.

Even with herbs and herbal supplements that are perfect for your system, there may be an initial period of reactivity or not feeling well. If there are extreme symptoms, stop taking the herbs or decrease the dosage. However, the belief that healing should automatically result in simply feeling better is incorrect. Symptoms like headaches, changes in bowel habits, fluctuations of energy or sleep, or even changes in mood can indicate that the body is shifting into a place of greater health. If the body is hyperreactive due to overwhelm, trauma, or autoimmunity, the initial response to favorable herbs can sometimes be negative. Such symptoms should disappear quite quickly (within a few days). If not, you may initially need the support of an experienced herbalist, who will be able to calm any fears as well as adjust herbal preparations and products as needed.

Ginger and Mint

People who have an overloaded nervous system or who are processing difficult energies through the digestive tract frequently experience nausea, dizziness, or an unsettled stomach.

There are two solutions to this that are quite easy to find in the local health food or grocery store: ginger for excess cold or mint for excess heat in the system. While the idea of therapeutic temperature may be a new concept for many of you, it is likely that through basic intuition either ginger or mint will feel correct for your digestive distress.

Ginger candies, or crystallized ginger, do have a bit of sugar added to them, but they are of immense benefit for cold or neutral types of nausea and digestive issues. While kundalini may feel quite hot, the area around the belly button will likely feel cool or cold to the touch; in such a case ginger is particularly indicated.

Ginger has the additional benefit of promoting circulation and helping with food stagnation (eating too much), especially after eating cold or damp foods (such as fried foods and dairy). It "wakes up" the digestive tract and works synergistically with kundalini. The Ayurvedic remedy Trikatu, a tablet that can be found in some health food stores, is typically a mixture of ginger, black pepper, and long pepper; it is an even hotter remedy, indicated for diets heavy in cold, damp foods (the person for whom this is indicated will often have a thick, greasy tongue coat).

Ginger root steeped in hot water with a bit of honey (real or raw honey, rather than synthetic honey) can be a wonderful way to start each morning, to invigorate the digestive tract. Using ginger to a greater degree in food preparations, such as the congee recipe, can be therapeutic. Masala chai tea drinks, which often contain ginger, may also be indicated.

The mint family is indicated for heat related nausea. Even basic mints from the grocery or convenience store can be of great assistance in cooling and restoring harmony to the digestive tract. Mint is especially indicated in the heat of summer to provide a cooling resource for the body, but can be used year-round as needed for digestive difficulties that include heartburn, constipation, or feelings of being irritated, either physically or emotionally.

Dandelion

Dandelion is particularly indicated for what is known as "liver excess": anger or bouts of rage, skin eruptions, poor digestion due to food retention or dietary excesses, hormonal issues, and water retention. It also provides a much needed bitter taste to our diets and lives, which has the effect of stimulating digestive secretions; the bile that is thus released breaks down fats and proteins in the body.

Dandelion leaves are loaded with nutrients, including vitamin C and potassium. However, it is important to note that dandelions in suburban or city settings may have been sprayed with chemicals, so be careful before picking any for your dinner.

Liquid extracts of dandelion are quite easy to find, especially in springtime when people seek to cleanse their systems. Instead of doing a fast and abrasive cleanse, start with 5-10 drops a day of liquid extracts (about half or a third of the dose that is recommended on most bottles) and build up week after week until digestion has improved, anger has lessened, and hormones have regulated.

Milk Thistle

Sometimes we tend to reach for aggressive cleanses and products that will produce large results or purge our systems in a noticeable way. But more often we require deep nurturing, rather than cleansing or purging of our systems, especially if we find ourselves preoccupied with ideas of being inwardly unclean, a sense of internal parasites that never clear, feelings of never being good enough, or a trauma history of not being nurtured appropriately, especially in early childhood.

Some consider milk thistle to be a liver cleanser, while in reality it can be seen as a liver nourisher that cleanses as a result of its nourishing actions. It is best used in tincture (liquid) form. It can gently rebuild the liver as well as restoring energetic reserves, moving energy through the digestive tract and body as a whole. It also gently harmonizes emotions, especially longstanding anger, passive-aggressive tendencies, depression and grief. Those who have issues with ragweed in their environment (such as hay fever) may have issues with milk thistle, but otherwise it is a gentle, powerful herb.

Valerian, Passionflower, and Skullcap

One of the more commonly known herbal products is valerian root, recognized for its ability to assist with sleep and insomnia and to decrease anxiety. Valerian has a sedative effect, and is indicated for people with high anxiety, emotional overwhelm, and difficulty falling asleep.

Passionflower is calming to the mind and spirit, but does not have the same degree of sedative effect as valerian (or valerian's side-effects of being groggy the next day or having an unsettled stomach). It is extremely gentle and nurturing, especially indicated for a restless mind and overthinking; it is gentle enough for even those with compromised systems to take. It is a powerful herbal ally to reach for in times of existential crisis, which can be combined with skullcap or utilized on its own for temporary emotional distress, difficulty sleeping, and mental overload.

Skullcap is another herb that is comforting, rather than tranquilizing. It promotes emotional well-being and relaxation, reduces inflammation and settles anxiety. Both skullcap and passionflower are known to be helpful when suffering from withdrawal from drugs or caffeine; they also help with emotional withdrawal from a relationship or marriage, and with anxiety that comes from moving or starting a new career. They are typically used for a short time, such as for a few weeks, rather than a few years.

Mushrooms and Reishi

While there are a wide variety of medicinal mushrooms, Reishi (or *Ling Zhi*) is particularly well known for its ability to boost the immune system, to build essence (or baseline energy) as well as to reinvigorate the system in times of significant depletion, such as chronic disease, long-term stress, chronic fatigue, and the after-effects of viral infections. It reduces stress by its ability to build up the baseline energy reserves of the body, and is known for its ability to promote longevity. It is also known as the "medicine of kings" for its ability to bestow vigor. In Chinese medicine, the dried mushroom is taken in teas or sprinkled on foods. Be careful to find a good source of Reishi through a reputable herbalist or long-standing herbal store; due to the interest in Reishi there are a variety of fakes as well as powders that may contain minimal amounts.

Ashwagandha

Ashwagandha has long been a staple of Ayurvedic medicine. It has seemingly opposing properties: it both calms anxiety, stress, and fear, and it invigorates those who are struggling with low energy and vitality.

Ashwagandha is known as an adaptogen; in simple terms this means that it builds up the person as a whole, and is specifically indicated for chronic diseases and long term issues. While members of the ginseng family (another herb that is used to restore vitality and energy) are often too hot and stimulating for those experiencing kundalini awakenings, the dual or opposing energies of ashwagandha mean that the nervous system is soothed as well as reinvigorated. This means that it can help reset long-term issues such as insomnia and poor sleep, or energy fluctuations and high stress.

As if this were not enough, it also supports the immune system, especially during times of immune distress, for example, during cancer treatments; it boosts the essence (or baseline energy of the body) to support a healthy reproductive tract and sexual function with issues such as lack of interest or performance difficulties.

It is typically used as a powder because it tastes rather foul. If there are autoimmune issues or difficulties with nightshades, ashwagandha may trigger reactions; it is best used in a formula that can be specifically balanced with other herbs by a competent herbalist and/or Ayurvedic practitioner.

Floradix

Floradix is a liquid supplement especially indicated for menstruating women to assist with iron deficiency. It is recommended over iron pills because due to its formulation it does not create constipation issues. Weakness during the menstrual cycle, dizziness, or blood clots (which can indicate difficulty with circulation and the production of blood), as well as more generalized signs of low energy, dark under-eye circles, cold hands and feet, and pain due to feelings of weak muscles point to symptoms that can be addressed by this supplement.

Trace Minerals

Trace minerals are essential minerals found in a large variety of foods. Due to the depletion of minerals from soil and our modern diet, we may not be getting all of the minerals that we need from the food that we eat. Trace minerals most effectively come through a liquid preparation added to water. Pills and pill casings are often difficult for compromised digestive tracts to absorb.

Trace minerals provide a large dose of magnesium, which people tend to lack, as well as selenium, iodine, calcium, zinc, and chloride, all of which help the mind and body perform well. Stress, lifestyle, and diet can deplete the nutritional and energetic reserves of the body, and trace minerals can be of great assistance in coming into nutritional and energetic balance.

Digestive Bitters

We lack bitter as a taste in most of our modern diets. While the idea of taking something bitter may not be appealing initially, the flavor of bitter strengthens digestive responses and allows for the flow of bile and digestive juices. Taking digestive bitters after a meal, especially if there is gas, bloating, heartburn, or other signs of indigestion, can allow for a reduction of symptoms.

Taking them over time, such as once a day, can encourage healthy bowel habits, support the digestive fire, cycle pancreatic and other digestive enzymes, and allow for a healthy liver, which helps us express emotions freely, particularly anger.

If there is significant digestive distress, start digestive bitters slowly and use only after meals. If there is significant nausea or a recent history of extreme digestive distress, such as vomiting after meals, digestive bitters may temporarily increase such symptoms, and so something like milk thistle or other herbs that increase energy and vitality should be used either first or in conjunction.

Herbal Infusions: Nettle and Oatstraw

One of the simplest methods of working with herbs is through infusions. These are teas that are brewed for long periods of time, and then drained and drunk on a daily basis. For this method of preparation, taught by herbalist Susun Weed, nettle leaf or oat straw stalk are suggested.

To make this preparation, put one ounce of the herb into a mason jar, pour hot water over the top, and replace the cap. Set this on the counter to steep anywhere from 5–10 hours. This results in a rich tea; strain it and drink the liquid portion. A typical dosage is to drink the entirety of the tea, but in the beginning split the liquid that comes from the one ounce of herbs into two doses; store the second dose in the refrigerator for the next day. It is suggested that the liquid be drunk in two days, otherwise the tea begins to break down.

These preparations are "simples"—use one herb at a time. Start with either nettle or oatstraw, depending on what you are struggling with. If you are female, I suggest beginning with nettle; although it can be used by both men and women, it is particularly good for women due to its iron content.

Nettle is an excellent nourishing herb that can be used long-term. It is high in calcium, iron, and other vitamins; because it is diuretic it assists in moving excess water through the body. There are not enough good things to say about nettle, as it is a powerful yet gentle ally to boost energy reserves and build vitality; it is a general tonic to which few people have any type of adverse reaction. Although it is an overall tonic, it is particularly aimed at the first and second chakra—the reproductive tract.

Oatstraw calms nervous stress, releases tension, and promotes healthy and resilient nervous and endocrine systems. Oatstraw is well known for its ability to "sow wild oats," reinvigorating the sex drive. It offers physical strength and mental clarity through gentle but profound nourishment for really anyone, but especially those who feel that their systems lack vitality and stability.

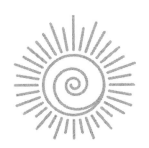

12

Finding Assistance

It is far more important to find a compassionate, experienced practitioner than one who practices a specific form of healing. That said, different modalities of healing target different aspects: some are more body oriented, while others may be body-mind, or energy-spirit oriented.

When choosing a practitioner, look for someone who has a decade of experience; this ensures that they have a wide range of direct experiences and a depth of knowledge that will be an asset in your own process. Otherwise, check their biography to see if they have any type of spiritual training or personal spiritual practice, which indicates a willingness to work with the spiritual layers of reality.

It is ideal that the practitioner practice whatever they are offering singularly and that they have credentials or certifications. In many of the massage and mind-spirit categories, practitioners may only need a weekend workshop in order to set up shop. That may be okay if that individual then has a decade of full-time practice and devotes themselves to personal study of their craft, but you do not want to be your practitioner's third client or even thirtieth, while you are going through something as complex as a kundalini awakening. Someone who offers thirty different types of bodywork is unlikely to have taken the time and focus to excel at one of them.

It is not essential that your practitioner has awakened kundalini, or even necessarily knowledge of spiritual awakenings. Of course that would be wonderful, but it is of far greater importance that the person you choose seems grounded, stable, and skillful. Most bodyworkers who have been in practice for longer than five years, and who have some awareness beyond the mere physical, will have experienced some of their clients doing spontaneous movements or shaking on the table.

What modality would be best for you really depends where you are in your process. However, there are some that may be contraindicated, or at least not recommended, during certain stages of the process. Below is a list of modalities and what they can offer for someone going through a kundalini awakening process.

Some people are still struggling with aspects of rugged individualism when it comes to spiritual awakening. This comes typically from a misunderstanding of personal responsibility—we may believe that we are to take on the world and our process alone. This may come from an isolating tendency arising out of trauma, where we have schismed from our communities and asking for support from one another.

Taking personal responsibility for ourselves includes the realization that we do not need to suffer alone; we often need help with our bigger blockages. We might struggle all on our own with something for six months, if not longer, when working with someone who could shift our process in a few sessions, if not a few minutes. We require another person to help us energetically shift larger patterns, otherwise we may feel like Atlas, struggling alone with the world on our shoulders.

We may also have some issues that simply require being witnessed by another person in order to heal. These could be big patterns of trauma, or they may simply be a small part of you that needs someone else's perspective. Or you may just need non-sexual compassionate touch. Our lack of touch, our disconnection from one another creates so much grief and pain. Learning that touch can be safe, and to allow another to nurture us, can allow us to work through many different types of trauma.

So many of us struggle needlessly because we do not know enough about holistic options, or prevent ourselves from seeing a counselor for talk therapy. I meet people who are truly drowning in their lives, yet they do not realize that reaching out for support is the greatest way of taking personal responsibility for ourselves. We all have varying degrees of trauma. There are many gifted healers out there, many of whom have courageously attended to their own deep processes, and who are more than willing to lead you through terrain they know well.

It is good to remember that experiencing this process, no matter how gradual, is traumatizing in and of itself. During times of trauma we tend to isolate; trauma in itself is an isolating, ungrounding process. And when we lack clarity and stability we may create beliefs that further disconnect us, taking us further away from health.

Some of the nervous system and physiological experiences that occur during the kundalini awakening process either need a very experienced teacher or a bodyworker versed in that type of work. If you are experiencing significant symptoms, I suggest visiting a practitioner for a series of treatment, perhaps ten sessions. This could be twice a week until symptoms are under control. For most, it will be once a week. Once distressing symptoms subside, typically appointments go down to once every other week, or once a month.

If you are more participatory and stable in your process, such as meditating daily, attending to your physical form with yoga or other flow-based exercise (such as martial arts, qi gong, or any form of activity that opens the joints of the body), or using sensory deprivation tanks, you may need fewer treatments, for instance, once a week or once a month. This would be to work with either anything significant that comes up, or for general balancing purposes.

Most practitioners have websites, or a bio or press release that will give you a decent impression of who they are and how they work. Nevertheless, you may need to try several practitioners before you find someone that you connect with and feel a deep synergy with. Someone may have all of the credentials in the world, but your personalities may not mesh well. Or they may be more versed in physical or sports medicine than working with energetically sensitive or spiritual patients.

In working with kundalini, it is important to keep in mind that treatments may not shift things right away, or there may be a difficult reaction after a session. The healing process does not automatically make us feel better. It may bring up a blockage of unresolved grief, release a muscle that causes us to feel sore the next day, or cause unprocessed traumatic memories to arise.

The Body Deva

I wrote *The Body Deva: Working with the Spiritual Consciousness of the Body* after going through my own kundalini awakening and educating myself rather endlessly in a variety of modalities, as well as working with clients for over a decade with the method.

The Body Deva is a method of self-inquiry as well as a form of healing that spans the spectrum of body-emotions-mind-spirit by rooting any pattern, from physical to spiritual, in the physical form. While I do recommend working in person with a practitioner, part of the reason that I developed this work is because people can be doing so much more and can be really empowered by deciding to take an active role in their own process.

There also may be understandable financial concerns that come with seeking treatment. It is recommended for people who are reasonably stable and who are ready to look within to resolve the issues, imbalances, and blockages in their lives. Taking responsibility for ourselves and our healing path is a big task. The Body Deva method requires some stability, as it asks you to reconsider beliefs.

This method of healing resolves anything and everything through the physical body to transform you on all levels of your being. It works with the understanding that what is preventing us from self-realization and liberation is the personal and collective trauma that we have experienced. We can then work with kundalini because it reveals the dysfunction in various parts of the body, different organs and the chakras. This method allows us to go into the body, to discover what trauma is being held in that area of the body and to release the held consciousness there.

During the awakening process it is important to have a process of self-inquiry. The Body Deva provides this method of internal questioning; it allows anyone to become more conscious about what is held within. This method can also be used to "speak" to kundalini itself, thus lessening many symptoms, basic reactivity, and resistance to the process.

CranioSacral Therapy

CranioSacral therapy is a light touch modality that works with the continuum of the sacrum, spinal cord, and skull, including the membranous structures that line the spinal canal and skull, osseous structures including the small bones that make up the skull and vertebrae, and the cerebrospinal fluid that flows through this continuum.

CranioSacral therapy provides care for imbalance at any level of the body—physical, mental/emotional, energetic and spiritual—and restores integrity and flow.

Since kundalini arises through the cerebrospinal matrix, and focuses on this continuum (although work may take place anywhere in the body) CranioSacral therapy is the ideal modality for those experiencing kundalini awakenings. It gently nourishes and decompresses the nervous system, reduces pain and encourages flow, all without putting additional stimulus into the body. It works with the rhythms and flows of the body as a whole, and considers the client as a whole person, rather than a mechanistic series of parts. Through this type of care, headaches may be treated in the hips or feet, or digestive disorders may find relief through restoring energetic and fluid flow through the brain.

SomatoEmotional release, or the processing of emotions and experiences through the physical form, can happen gently and safely with an experienced therapist. Trauma care is done in a gentle yet profound way, and the focus on meeting clients where they are (rather than pushing them in any way) and meeting the system where it is, allows the often hyperreactive nervous system or trauma response in the body to gently release on its own terms.

Additionally, some CranioSacral therapists work intraorally (in the mouth and around the throat) or viscerally (with the organs of the body). They may also use other modalities alongside, including Zero Balancing or Lymphatic Drainage.

Experienced CranioSacral therapists are used to their clients shaking, performing automatic body movements, and having emotional releases; they know how to work with traumatized populations and with chronic or mysterious health conditions. Some of the most irritating physiological issues that arise from the kundalini awakening process, such as muscle fasciculations along the spine, can be resolved by a competent CranioSacral therapist.

CranioSacral therapy in its purest intent is the ability to meet people with neutrality, and to work with whatever arises. Experienced Cranio-Sacral therapists who are versed in mind-body-spirit and have a decade of experience are worth their weight in gold. However, like many things that seek to become more mainstream, it is typical to find people who have taken a weekend workshop in CranioSacral therapy, who do it infrequently, or who seek to reduce the modality to a linear, technical and non-spiritual form of bodywork. Look for someone who focuses on CranioSacral therapy in their practice, and who is certified or well studied in the modality.

Yoga

Yoga is another modality that has gained huge popularity in the West, and teachers can range from devoting their lives to the practice to attending a quick course and gaining certification. If there is a yoga teacher in your area who has devoted their lives to immersive study, both intellectual as well as practical, their guidance can be invaluable. Yogis who are competent and experienced can guide you towards greater physical health, ensure that energy cycles properly through the meridians of the body, and teach breath-work practices in a comprehensive way.

As with many modalities imported into the West, the philosophical, spiritual, and energetic understandings of yoga have been all but elimi-nated. Yoga has been turned from a spiritual science into physical exercise. Look for a teacher who has a comprehensive background in yoga or has studied in depth, and who seems grounded and vibrant. Many yoga teachers offer individual sessions where they can evaluate your body and its needs, providing individual instruction to open up the static or held energies of the body.

While it may seem that Kundalini yoga would be the correct choice for those experiencing a kundalini awakening, practices such as the breath of fire and using a heated room tend to exacerbate symptoms. Generally the most helpful forms of yoga for clients over the years have been either *yin yoga*, basic *hatha yoga*, or if there is a focus on creating strength and stability in the system, *Iyengar yoga*. If there is injury or weakness of the physical form, many yoga studios have *restorative* types of yoga, which use chairs, props, and pillows to ensure that no further injury takes place. Static poses rather than flow-based practices allow proper time for the joints to open and for energetic flow to occur, including the flow of kundalini.

Ayurveda

The largest benefit of Ayurveda for kundalini awakenings is that practi-tioners have an understanding of kundalini energy; they have treatment protocols for those who are having difficulties with the process.

Having an understanding of sushumna, ida, and pingala, as well as kundalini, can be of immense support to anyone actually going through the process. To have a medicine that discusses chakra and energetic imbalances, as well as specific considerations for when the process has gone awry, can be crucial for anyone in a spiritual awakening process.

Many who study Ayurveda also have knowledge of yoga and yogic philosophy, as well as a comprehensive understanding of dietary, medita-tive, and lifestyle considerations. The practitioner will discuss your sleep, sexual habits, spiritual history, emotional history, and any physical concerns in depth. This indicates your "type" and what course of treatment would be best for you. Ayurveda is particularly strong with digestive issues; most practitioners will be able to work with emotional overwhelm, upheaval, and spiritual experiences, as long as the client is not in crisis mode. A series of sessions is often required.

One of the most helpful treatments for those experiencing pre-kundalini or kundalini awakening is Panchakarma. This is a series of three to five treatments that release stagnant energy, or energy that has become out of balance due to excesses or imbalanced approaches to diet, lifestyle, sexual habits, or thought. Subsequent treatments focus on rebalancing the system; you will receive lifestyle and diet instruction suitable for your unique constitution.

The problem, as it always is in the modern world, is that it doesn't take that much effort or depth to receive a certificate in Ayurveda. Look for someone who has engaged in immersive study, and who has devoted a great deal of time and energy to their craft.

One of the difficulties with Ayurveda is that it has been turned into a spa treatment. The oil treatments certainly feel good, and are relaxing, but "holistic" treatments in the West can be very superficial. There are practitioners who are not yet conscious of things like spiritual experiences, or who may not have any type of energetic sensitivity.

However, if you find a Ayurvedic practitioner who has devoted a great deal of time and effort, over five or ten years, chances are they will have the experience of working with kundalini awakenings and spiritual imbalances; their treatments will be specifically geared towards those with complex or multi-faceted difficulties.

Zero Balancing

Zero Balancing is a method of gentle body work that focuses on the energetics of bones, as well as the energetic currents that run through the deeper layers of the body. Its specific protocol works with the joints and areas where bones articulate with one another, which is where energy tends to stagnate.

This modality is performed with gentle touch on a massage table. The participant is clothed and experiences different body parts being held, range of motion of joints to find energetic stagnation or improper articulation, and gentle finger pressure to release. In each session the practitioner discusses a "frame," or what the client wants out of the session—physically, emotionally, energetically, and spiritually.

Zero Balancing is a spiritual modality that works with the deeper energetics of the body, promoting profound and gentle change in its vibratory nature. It is nurturing and incredibly grounding. There is specific attention paid to the pelvis, the rib cage, and the feet that provides for energetic releases that are hard to find through any other modality.

Due to the nature of the work, many Zero Balancers are energetically sensitive and spiritually in tune; they also possess deep knowledge of the physical structure of the body. This work provides grounding, embodiment, and gentle release in a contained way: releases are met energetically by the practitioner through what is known as "interface," or meeting the person the way donkeys do when they lean into one another. This type of interface allows for feelings of safety as well as even larger releases of energy to cycle gently, instead of creating further trauma, confusion, or chaos for the body.

Zero Balancing is especially indicated for physical issues, for grounding and embodiment issues, and for imbalances of a deep or existential spiritual nature (such as belief systems, ancestral energies, or existential depression). Look for someone who is certified or has taken multiple courses and is an active presence in the Zero Balancing community.

Hakomi

Hakomi is a word that means: "How do you stand in relation to these many realms?" It is a form of body psychotherapy, or in simpler terms, a healing method for trauma that understands that trauma and emotions are held within the physical form. Through gentle touch, word prompts, and gentle movement, a practitioner finds how trauma manifests through the physical form, and uncovers the beliefs or organizing systems that it has created in your life.

This method requires a bit of intuition and the ability to look deep within the client to see what is organizing their reality. We tend to swim on the surface of things, and do not care to look towards the ocean floor. But it is by working at that ocean floor that we can drastically shift how we look at the world, what we believe is possible for ourselves in this world, and improve our health. We all carry so much trauma, and the engaged method of healing that Hakomi offers approaches trauma in a way that is both gentle and profound. Many of its practitioners have seen and heard all sorts of stories, and are used to things like automatic body movements, shaking, emotional releases, as well as the worst sorts of trauma that this world unfortunately visits upon so many of us.

Hakomi practitioners are typically certified after going through a multi-year program, and most practitioners of this modality are either therapists or highly experienced bodyworkers. It is recommended for trauma release, and for those willing to explore their "ocean floor."

Spiritual Healing (Shamanic Healing)

Spiritual healers have the ability to navigate between many realms for the good of their communities, or for individual clients. Ideally spiritual healers (or shamanic practitioners) have the natural sight and aptitude to be able to interface with the natural world, spiritual realms, and this world, and they have gone through an intensive training process or apprenticeship. A spiritual healer who has been in full-time practice for a decade or more is ideal. This ensures that they have the experience to resolve even the most complex of issues.

There is a profound schism in the modern world between ourselves and the spiritual realms. Unfortunately many spiritual and shamanic practitioners rely on mental and thought-based practices rather than spiritual work, and do not have clear enough perspective to see the layers of reality. Neither discernment nor aptitude are tested for in this work, and there is no real certification to enter this field. This means that frequently ethics, professional practices, and other important issues are not a part of training for spiritual practitioners.

The training to become a spiritual worker is long. It typically involves five years or more of focus on personal healing along with a decade long apprenticeship with a competent teacher. It is necessary to move beyond personal wounding to be able to hold power as well as to not be reactive to clients who are often emotionally volatile or in significant distress.

The spiritual healer must have clear sight; this cannot happen if someone is seeing through the lens of fractured thoughts, through mental-emotional imbalances, or who lacks grounding or functioning in this world. Spiritual workers typically spend decades cultivating spiritual relationships that allow them to gather information and work in the spiritual and natural realms.

An excellent spiritual worker is somewhat rare, but it is important to seek them out. Ancestral healing, trauma healing, past life healing, release of energies that may impact the body, as well as spiritual understandings and guidance, are part of what they have to offer. If you go to an authentic spiritual worker, do not expect to be coddled, or to have your illusions agreed with. Their job is to assist you by shifting the spiritual dynamics of your case, which then creates profound physical, emotional, and mental shifts. This is done by mediating or navigating among forces within you, between you and the natural world, and between you and the spiritual realms.

Spiritual workers frequently do divination to see if they can be of assistance to you. Many spiritual workers do work via distance, and since the focus is on the spiritual layers and dynamics, it does not matter much to a competent practitioner whether the session takes place in person or via distance.

Ayahuasca, Marijuana, and Plant Medicines

To many who revere and work with the consciousness of the vine, ayahuasca is referred to as *Mother Kundalini*. It can provide purgation (purification) of the body as well as experiences of heightened consciousness. Done humbly with a competent shaman, ayahuasca can be a catalyst to profound realizations and expanded consciousness.

If someone is stuck in the purification process, ayahuasca can provide immense healing and processing of energies. However, many people blame ayahuasca when difficult emotions and processing experiences occur (similar to meditation). We always look to solve our issues simply and with no discomfort; we simply wish to feel better, and if we do not feel good immediately we at least wish to be anesthetized or feel numb. Ayahuasca is not about a quick fix, getting high, or someone or something else doing the work for us. But if we realize that this type of healing means traversing and processing what is held within, in the care of a spiritual worker who has a profound connection and calling to work with ayahuasca, we can have an invaluable and transformative experience.

It is important to properly educate oneself, understand the benefits of working with such a consciousness, and attend to recommended diets for the sort of purgation and processing that are part of working with ayahuasca. This ensures humility and transformation of large blockages. Integration after such experiences occurs through spiritual work or with an understanding therapist who has knowledge or is willing to learn about plant medicines.

Due to romanticization we believe that ayahuasca will solve all issues within a single session, but even powerful medicines take time and effort.

The spirit of marijuana can ease pain, resolve digestive issues, and transform consciousness. However, marijuana is a fire spirit (no matter the method of delivery) and stoking the fires of kundalini can lead to evolution of consciousness. It can also lead to overuse over time, diminishing the body's natural fire, including kundalini. However, light to moderate usage can be quite helpful especially in place of pain medications and antidepressants or other pharmaceuticals.

Substance abuse can be a factor as marijuana is fairly readily available, and people understandably look to numb painful emotions. While such numbing may be necessary or helpful in certain cases, ideally the spirit of the plant and its abilities to stoke fire with moderate usage can be of assistance, rather than another thing in this world that skews the mind or dampens or distracts the soul.

Marijuana usage can also mimic some of the signs of kundalini awakening without any type of actual emergence of the energy. In such cases, abstract thought would be heightened, as would other symptoms of being high, but long-term transformation of consciousness would not occur.

There is a wide variety of other substances, including LSD and mushrooms, that can foster the transformation of consciousness. For those looking to evolve or participate in their own transformation process, it is important to realize that such medicines bring out the inherent potential of the system, and are a teacher and guide, rather than an external object to imbibe or get high from. Such medicines are in no way necessary for enlightenment, but can be a profound ally in the process if approached correctly.

Castellino Pre- and Perinatal Work

We hold so much unprocessed trauma in regards to our entering this world. Anything from what our mothers ate to how they were emotionally feeling to whether they wanted us or not makes a profound energetic impact on how we relate to the world.

Traditional psychology is not adept at addressing experiences in utero and in infancy and early childhood (preverbal states). This is because they are not states of mental or verbal reasoning or conscious awareness.

Healing of in utero trauma often results in profound shifts in consciousness, and an understanding of why and how you operate in the world. We create our deepest blueprints for our stance in the world in the womb and in very early infancy. If we did not get the emotional, spiritual, or nutritional nurturing that we needed in utero, we will continually experience that lack in the outer world until it is healed.

The way that we enter this world can also leave an incredible imprint on us; by resolving any trauma related to whether we, or others involved with the birth process (mother, father, partner, extended family) were excited or fearful, uncertain or not wanting our presence, we can find ourselves relating to the world much differently. This work is also helpful for those who were adopted, abandoned, or born through a surrogate, because feelings of being lost, traumatized, or unrooted are very common in this population.

Practitioners of Castellino Prenatal and Birth Therapy can be difficult to find. Many of them are trained in biodynamic CranioSacral therapy, or other types of bodywork that have deep understandings of the fluid systems of the body, as well as the energetics and spiritual nature of the physical form.

In utero work can also be facilitated to some degree through flotation tanks, through water work where a bodyworker may do CranioSacral therapy, shiatsu, or other movement therapies in a pool, or through some spiritual workers, specifically ones that work with The Body Deva. If you have the chance to work with someone with this specific of training, no matter where you are in your process, I would highly recommend doing so. Releasing base patterning that has organized your whole existence can result in big leaps in healing, as well as greater consciousness overall.

Many practitioners who do this type of work have the compassion and sensitivity to work with a wide degree of difficulties, and even fairly emotionally fragile or traumatized clients.

Thai Bodywork and Shiatsu

Thai bodywork and shiatsu are both forms of bodywork that focus on moving energy through the meridians, the activation of specific points in the body, and pressure on specific areas of the body to harmonize and cycle energy. They are typically done clothed, on a mat on the floor. Although some forms of tabletop work are taught, I would highly recommend someone who does work on a mat. This is not only because such individuals are more likely to be highly trained, but because if you find or have concerns that bodywork will cause you to go into spontaneous body positions, hand positions, or shaking, receiving treatment on a mat on the floor is likely to be perfect for you.

Thai bodywork is popularly referred to as "assisted yoga." The therapist moves your body into varying yoga positions, and applies pressure in varying ways to move energy along the meridians ("sen lines" or energy channels of the body). This can be a tremendous asset to someone who is suffering from physical pain, or who is a bit later in their process and finds themselves stuck and unable to process a trauma that is coming up due to restrictions in their physical form.

Thai bodywork is typically meant for people who are reasonably healthy, and who are emotionally-mentally stable enough to be able to have moderate to large energetic or emotional releases.

We may have an ongoing problem, a "loop" that we cannot seem to break down, or an emotion or trauma that we simply cannot fully process. We get stuck because our bodies are stuck. It is by opening up the joints in the body, receiving help for our bodies to achieve a state of greater flow, that whatever we are stuck in can move, change, and shift. It would likely be unable to do so if we had not received a session to physically open our neck, or our legs, or whatever is physically in pain or blocked within us.

Thai bodywork can be quite strong, and while some therapists are more sensitive, many of them can be quite sports medicine or physically oriented. Such individuals are an asset on our path, as they look at things from another perspective. Many Thai bodywork practitioners are also yogis, and so they may have practices that can help you ground, embody, or stabilize your system. I do not suggest receiving this form of bodywork if you are dealing with overwhelm, particularly emotional overwhelm, or if your body is depleted to the point that it requires nurturing.

Shiatsu involves movement of the physical form on a mat and is typically more gentle than Thai bodywork. If you ever have the opportunity to participate in water-based shiatsu, where the work is done in a pool, it is simply incredible, especially since kundalini in its "free" state is very much a feeling and expression of flow, quite similar to the flow of water.

A shiatsu session involves finger pressure on acupuncture points or energy centers of the body, light stretching, and various types of massage. Many shiatsu therapists have expertise in how to work with the abdomen. If you have digestive complaints, the type of energetic centering and realignment that shiatsu can offer is quite helpful.

Most shiatsu therapists have experience with emotional release, however it is best to be at a point where you are not drowning in your process. Shiatsu is a good example of a type of work that spans the spectrum; it is very much physically oriented, opens up the joints and areas of the body where energy stagnates, but it also has an appreciation and understanding of mind, body, and emotions. Many shiatsu practitioners may also have a spiritual outlook, which brings the work into the full spectrum of mind-body-spirit.

Rolfing

Rolfing and Structural Integration practitioners look at how the body is organized in gravity. Their purpose, through a series of 10 or 12 sessions, is to realign the body, specifically the fascia (the body stocking) to reduce pain, open up the musculature, and to facilitate the flow of energy and fluids throughout the body.

We rarely recognize how tangled we are; we may not recognize how something like fascia can contribute to a wide range of dysfunctions within the body. When we are traumatized or have held emotions, they are often sectioned off within a part of our bodies. Our physical bodies organize around this weakness and fracturing, causing the physical body to be out of alignment, weak, and in pain.

We also may have physical experiences, for example, car accidents or daily lifestyle issues such as sitting for long periods of time, that result in our bodies not being physically and energetically balanced.

Most Rolfers are very well trained, with an in-depth knowledge of anatomy and physiology. Some have taken additional training in assessing the movement of the body; they may have their clients walk to see where energy and structure is static. There are also some Rolfers who have taken CranioSacral or other trainings so that they can work with a continuum of healing, and with any energetic or emotional releases that may occur as a result of manipulating the deep structures of the human form.

Rolfing is particularly indicated for pain patterns, and does have a focus on the physical form. A series of sessions is required so that balance can be created in gravity for the entirety of the human body. We are a complex system of pulleys and levers, tissues and muscles that work together to ensure physical balance. The work can be somewhat painful or intense, even for those who have a decent capacity to handle life stresses and are balanced emotionally. However, it is indicated for several reasons. In general I suggest that someone get a "ten series" about once a decade if they are able to, as our bodies do get out of alignment with gravity and this results in a wide range of dysfunction and disorders, including, unexpectedly, digestive and menstrual issues.

Without a properly aligned physical structure, kundalini awakening may exacerbate imbalances within the physical structure. It does not have the ability to awaken and flow, or to release the held emotional or trauma-based material that has been sectioned off and held by the physical structure unless the physical structure is realigned and opened.

Some Rolfers also have the ability to do intraoral work and intranasal work; the mouth and nose hold a tremendous amount of structural imbalance as well as energetic and emotional holding, and to experience release through skilled touch of these areas is quite profound.

Rolfing is suggested for stable, reasonably healthy individuals; it is particularly indicated for pain, but is also suggested for those later in their process who are able and willing to work with their process, and are looking to move into greater states of consciousness by finding and releasing what is held within the tissues and joints of the body.

Acupuncture

Acupuncture is a part of Traditional Chinese Medicine (TCM), whose practitioners are educated in acupuncture, bodywork and techniques such as moxibustion, gua sha, and cupping. Many have also been trained in herbalism, diet and nutrition, meditation or martial arts, as well as varying forms of bodywork and energy work.

For pain syndromes, digestive issues, and emotional regulation, acupuncture and Chinese medicine provide immense benefit. Acupuncture rebalances and moves energy through the channels of the body, so there can be proper flow, as well as balance.

An acupuncturist looks at your tongue and feels your pulse, both of which provide a map of the body and how you are doing overall. I recommend an individual appointment, or a private one, instead of community acupuncture where many individuals are worked with simultaneously. This ensures that the practitioner takes a full history and is attuned to the complexity of presentation.

Acupuncture can be quite strong, so it can be hard for extremely depleted patients or those who are very sensitive to energy. Approaches like moxibustion and diet can certainly be done to boost energy. But until the energy reserves of the body are filled up a bit more, it is best to use gentler forms of acupuncture, like Japanese or Toyohari acupuncture, which feature gentler techniques, working energetically with needles instead of inserting them into the meridians of the body. Practitioners with training in varying types of acupuncture will often list them on their website, or you can simply ask if they have experience working with sensitive or energetically depleted systems.

Chiropractic

Chiropractic can be quite helpful for kundalini awakenings, especially if kundalini is stuck at a physical juncture in the spine and requires physical manipulation to flow better energetically.

Look for someone who has studied chiropractic or osteopathic care in the "old school" (or who is interested in the mind-body-spirit continuum as evidenced through their studies and other certifications). Alternatively, Network Chiropractic, which is a much gentler and more energetic form of chiropractic care, and similar forms can be quite helpful for those experiencing kundalini awakenings.

Early chiropractic understandings included the energetic and spiritual significance of the spine and skull. However, many chiropractors these days tend to be focused on sports medicine, or may lack any type of knowledge of issues related to spirituality, energy, or emotional imbalances.

Some chiropractors also offer a large variety of supplements, even to sensitive patients who may need simpler forms of care or lower dosages of vitamins, herbs, or minerals. Those experiencing kundalini who have compromised digestion may be unable to absorb pills or capsules, so liquids are often necessary, with a regimen focused on one or two supplements at a time.

A good chiropractor is like a gem, incredibly useful to those with any type of physical pain, including internal discomforts. Some are incredibly knowledgeable about nutrition, or can give advice regarding diet and lifestyle. Ask if they use less forceful adjustments, and if they have training in energy work or any type of personal spiritual cultivation.

Naturopathic

Naturopaths go through a multi-year course of study and licensure in diet, herbal, as well as allopathic study (Western medicine). They typically form a bridge between allopathy and practices like folk medicine, which focus on herbology and lifestyle.

A naturopath will be able to read and understand your blood test from your doctor, as well as recommend specific herbs and supplements for anxiety, digestive issues, fatigue, and other internal physiological and emotional imbalances.

Finding a naturopath who has any spiritual knowledge or ability to understand or appreciate spiritual issues might be somewhat difficult. There is also a tendency to offer a large array of supplements, vitamins, or other regimens that may be unnecessary or too difficult for a sensitive or reactive system to take in.

However, naturopaths who have extensive experience and a compassionate, client-focused disposition can be invaluable for finding a balance between holistic and allopathic care, figuring out complex digestive disorders, evaluating complex internal medicine cases, and prescribing proper nutrition for your system.

Psychotherapy

There is an inherent difficulty in the psychotherapeutic evaluation and treatment of kundalini in that it is not just a mental and emotional event. Certainly psychological material is unearthed and cleared in the purification process, and processing of the impact of early childhood and adolescent trauma is hugely important. But without treatment of the physiology, especially the nervous system, fascia, and cerebrospinal fluid flow, those with kundalini awakenings will not find relief in psychotherapy alone.

In addition, enmeshment in the mind-body paradigm means that therapists are looking for pathologies or imbalances. The normalcy that practitioners are wanting to establish in clients, by the very nature of their diagnostic criteria, is one that—I will say this gently—is not preferable for anyone who is reasonably conscious.

However, some practitioners have immersed themselves in spiritual traditions, shamanism, bodywork, or other methods that understand that the mind and body are not separate. Those in transpersonal, Jungian, or existential fields of psychotherapy are the most inclined to look at the spiritual process as one of deep inquiry and personal transformation, rather than a pathological one.

Talk therapy can be an incredible asset, especially when processing during the first phase. If we have completely isolated ourselves due to trauma, including the trauma of spiritual awakening itself, talk therapy is essential to open us up to grounding in the world and connecting with people again.

Look for a therapist with a good head on their shoulders, who focuses on offering tools and building emotional intelligence. If we are no longer capable of functioning, or suffering from significant trauma and emotional-mental distress to the point that we are no longer participating in communal reality, or may be a danger to ourselves or others, therapists have the tools and education to offer care ethically and appropriately. If we are in a state of overwhelm or unable to traverse the process, then medication or hospitalization may become necessary, and a compassionate therapist can be an important ally.

We have a great deal of stigma regarding unseen illnesses, ones that we cannot put a microscope on. Mental illness should be seen similarly to physical illness: many conditions can be helped or even healed by holistic, energetic, or spiritual methods of care or bodywork, but some will not. Stopping the kundalini process through the use of medications is always something to consider. Though it may be difficult to come off such medications, they can be life-saving, and there should be no stigma in taking them. Of course, it should not be the first approach, and only after careful consideration with a competent therapist—not a general physician.

As with many practitioners, check to see what types of training they have done, what their specialties and interests are. Many will offer a brief phone call or email interaction to see how they may be of service. I suggest going for at least three sessions before deciding if they are the right person for you; it may take a bit of time to find someone who resonates with you personally and who is open to spiritual experiences.

What to Look for in a Spiritual Teacher

There is a long list of what to look for in a spiritual teacher: humility, continual exploration and evolution of their own consciousness, stillness, and the willingness to point students inward, among others.

An authentic spiritual teacher is humbled by the vastness of the cosmos. They have deepening knowledge when it comes to their own path; any direct experience and unfolding into greater consciousness only expands the more conscious they are. Someone who is becoming more conscious will have new teachings, a new way of being, or new depths to add as a result of their own, direct experiences.

Direct experience allows for nuance, for the movement from intellectualism into a space of direct gnosis. While many spiritual experiences are simply ineffable, a good spiritual teacher meets students where they are. They may describe things in the language of a kindergartener or with the utmost simplicity to someone at the beginning of their path. They may go into more intellectual conversations with an intellectual or philosopher who lacks direct experience. With their most advanced students, they may simply sit in silence, or work with symbols or states that require a high level of consciousness. Any spiritual teacher worth their salt is someone who points out the blind spots in their students to help their growth. They do not participate in the projections or "plays" of their students—the roles and "loops" and illusory chaos that those individuals bring.

Many seekers wish to move past foundational knowledge to the most experienced and advanced practices, not understanding that foundational knowledge is what allows for those advanced practices to be something more than just imaginings of the mind. A spiritual teacher focuses on foundational practices, even with their advanced students, to ensure a healthy balance of mind, body, and spirit.

Look for a spiritual teacher who has educated themselves with sincerity and depth. This means cultivation over years, decades, and even lifetimes. While some teachers make claims that can be understandably hard to see through, a spiritual teacher should be able to have an in-depth conversation about their spiritual path and what they have studied.

If someone has studied allopathic medicine, psychology, or other modalities this does not mean that they have studied spiritual viewpoints. These individuals can offer a helpful first step, especially if you are looking for stepping stones to a spiritual path.

You may come across people who believe that their mental and emotional fracturing mean that they are great shamans, prophets, or teachers; they rarely see that such imbalances should be worked with and healed. Someone who is in an imbalanced state will have difficulty providing any help to others seeking stability or higher consciousness.

There are also seekers who find teachers who simply mirror their own wounds; they find someone who is broken the same way they are, such as both having wounded five year-olds within. What is wounded within us seeks to replay the same "loops" again and again. It is only by becoming conscious of them that we can find a teacher who will lead us forward, instead of catering to our wounds.

It is always a question of whether we are being led by our wounds or by what is unhealed within us. Are we looking for someone who is more than willing to accept our projected guru inclinations, so we can give away our power to them? Ideally, we are being led to someone who can point us inward, who can show us clarity, who can help us to see our blind spots.

A realized spiritual teacher has an immense amount of stillness—a state of grace, in which one realizes with humility a state of flow, compassion, and grounding within the physical form. A teacher who has a sense of humor, and a degree of lightness, is also something to look for, as they realize the cosmic joke and playfulness of the Universe. A good teacher will not be perfected, but very human, and willing to clearly see their very human imperfections. So many wounded individuals balk at any sign of imperfection, preferring their teachers to wear masks or to live up to a romanticized ideal.

It is sadly true that there is much superficiality, illusion, and lack of regard for spirit in spiritual teachers these days. Yet there are also wonderful spiritual teachers out there. They may not be as loud. They do not need to be. It may feel impossible to find someone who has devotion, education, and direct experience of the spiritual path. But if you are willing to recognize that the spiritual path requires effort, cultivation, and devotion, and you are looking for clarity rather than to perpetuate illusion or wounded states, you will find the right spiritual teacher for you.

The Light at the End of the Tunnel

Many years ago I was reading a book by the author Ophiel in which he likens the process of writing a book to an exorcism. This work has been the encapsulation of many years' effort, an obsessive search and education process that has allowed me to simply convey what I have learned. To talk about this process and its hardships, as well as its benefits, with clarity and authenticity, or as much as I am able to provide at this time.

In many ways the end of the path signifies an end to a period of time, a death and opportunity for rebirth. In this book I hope that I have forwarded the consideration of spiritual awakenings and kundalini so that they can be taken seriously in this world. So the process can be clearly understood, so those who wish to support others while going through this process can distinguish who may need an experienced yogi and who may benefit from talk therapy.

I hope to create a baseline, and in so doing to encourage those who can recognize themselves in these pages to know that there are others out there like themselves, and to be willing to accept support. It is beyond time that we have a nuanced view of spiritual awakening in the modern world. It is our birthright, not a pathology. It is an evolution of the soul, a call to greater being. The modern world has little place for magic, for spirit, and for direct spiritual revelation. We have relegated such things to pathological or psychological aberrations. Let us see them instead as leading to an evolution of human consciousness, greater stability, humility, and compassion, to an increased interest in being of benefit to the world.

I truly believe that any evolution within myself has occurred because I have always been willing to look towards what is immensely and unmistakably human within me.

Long ago, I realized that the notion of perfection was a mask, an illusion that is perpetuated in the modern world because we hope for such illusions. We hope to be free of pain, to have someone give us all the answers. It was incredibly freeing for me to recognize that those who are the most realized are the most human. They will freely say that they do not know; they will openly state what their imperfections are. It is by grounding in this deep humanity, rather than looking towards the mask of perfection, that we can release ourselves from this pervasive illusion.

Other necessary traits include openness, curiosity, a deep yearning to find something larger than the self, and perhaps most importantly, the ability to see beyond the wounded ego-mind, which is always seeking to keep us who we are and how we are. Authenticity and fortitude are always a part of any dedicated spiritual path.

I am reminded of the cartoon with two booths: one with a banner that says "pleasant illusions" and the other that says "complex truths." We know which booth most of us will be crowded around. People who visit that other booth are the ones who awaken.

It is by looking within, and directly at the parts of ourselves that suffer, at what is not working in our lives, and at the aspects of ourselves that may be at that first booth that we liberate ourselves. Such a journey is treacherous, although it has great rewards.

In my meditations lately I have been sitting with the aspect of myself that is wondering if such a journey is truly worthwhile. Beyond illusion, kundalini awakening and spiritual awakening is a path of hardship. It is a path of immense difficulty, and one that takes tremendous fortitude to traverse. Despite so many moments of beauty and wonder, so much healing and evolution, it is a path of enormous responsibility. It is a path that is carved out by daily, lived experience. Of looking directly at what is not working in our lives, of looking at what is false, of looking at the outer world to see what needs to be healed within. Such a path can be wearing over time, despite its incredible rewards. This is one of the many paradoxes of this journey—the recognition of the simultaneous hardship and beauty of such an experience.

The answer that came forward in my meditation was that this hard task is, in fact, the reason that we are here, and this is why it is worth it. We are here to evolve, to become. It is so easy to look towards the illusions because they give us permission to stay who and what we are. We love the idea of knowing what is unknowable with finality, to believe in the Western myth of progress and exceptionalism that gives rise to the rugged individualist who always seeks to be superior to his fellow man, who seeks to dominate the forces within and without.

We love the myth of simplicity, of simple rules and guidelines that we can follow to be deemed "good." That can allow for us to perpetuate the superiority/inferiority loop: the idea that we are in any way superior to our fellow human beings due to ideology or way of being. The idea that we can have mastery, or even knowledge, about what is ultimately ineffable. We offer our power and capacity to spiritual teachers who claim mastery, complete knowledge, and perfection, who give us guidelines and tell us who we should be.

If there were one simple piece of advice that I would offer about finding a teacher, or about how to not get stuck in the process yourself, it would be to look towards your humanity. You do not need to be perfect. Perfection is a mask, it is an illusion, and the experience of infinity destroys any need to be anything other than who you are right now. The experience of infinity, even for a moment, reveals that we can only know a tiny corner of the Cosmos, no matter how realized we are. That nobody has all of the answers. That we are all evolving, even in realized and enlightened states. We all have more to learn, more to discover, more ability to evolve into the vastness of infinity. The more we experience such vastness, the more humility we have, the less masterful we feel. Those who have discovered this are the teachers to look for, and the quality that will show anyone that they have attained a perspective that is worth listening to. Look towards any parts of yourself that seek to be superior or separate from others—they will show you what aspects are not conscious or whole. Look at what qualities or people you or others continually point to in the outer world—this shows you the greatest blind spots of what needs to be healed within.

The spiritual awakening process is a breakdown of belief, a breakdown of these masks and illusions. It is a breakdown of the myth of the individual, of knowledge, of mastery. It is a deconstruction process that allows for what is real and true to emerge. For a focus on humanity, a recognition of how little time we have within our human forms and how precious our connections are. It is not a looking away or a denial of the human form, the senses, or any of our experiences here. We are within human forms for a reason: within our human forms we have an ability to evolve that is not afforded to us in other states. We are intended to evolve through our physical forms, not separate from them. In our short period of time that we are humans, we always have a choice of whether we are going to look within or not, to look towards our wounds or perpetuate them. It is a daily, hourly, and even momentary choice of whether we are going to separate or connect, to perpetuate what is wounded within us, or to heal.

It is a choice to look towards all aspects of ourselves as a source of beauty. It is by seeing even the darkest aspects of ourselves as worthy of compassion that we can change. It is by allowing what is unhealed and thus disconnected within us to have its voice that it can heal. Such disconnected aspects within us will not heal by being bullied, called wrong, or told that they need to be love and light. It is by seeing our imperfections as beauty that we can see them embodying as much light as even the greatest aspects of hope and love within ourselves.

There are many beautiful teachings out there, many competent teachers. These are keys that will allow for you to unlock depths in your own spiritual path. The spiritual path is a deeply individual one, even as there are commonalities that can be pointed at. Nobody else can make the journey for you. As Krishnamurti once famously said, "In oneself lies the whole world and if you know how to look and learn, the door is there and the key is in your hand. Nobody on earth can give you either the key or the door to open, except yourself."

Through this book, through my explorations and experiences and study, I hope that I have offered you a key to find that doorway within yourself. To find authenticity, to find meaning, to find your way beyond all of the captivating and glittery illusions that are so prevalent in this world.

There is a light at the end of the tunnel, and it is a continual evolution of self, a freeing of self of the beliefs and traumas and societal constraints that once held you in captivity. Wherever you are in your spiritual awakening process, know that the light is there. And it is beautiful.

Further Reading

For further information, I offer a curriculum of study. This booklist is separated into five sections; books from section three, four, or five may not be fully understood if books from sections one and two are not read first. Being in a later section does not indicate that a book is necessarily of more worth, but simply that you may need a background in the previous sections in order to understand it fully.

These books are chosen either because they helped me tremendously on my own path, or because I respect them as gatekeepers to deeper layers of knowledge.

SECTION ONE

Awakening: A Sufi Experience by Pir Vilayat Inayat Khan; TarcherPerigee, 2000

Cutting through Spiritual Materialism by Chogyam Trungpa; Shambhala, 2002

God Spoke to Me by Eileen Caddy; Findhorn Press, 1992

Kundalini, Evolution and Enlightenment edited by John White; Paragon House, 1998

Spiritual Emergency: When Personal Transformation Becomes A Crisis by Stanislav Grof; TarcherPerigee, 1989

Stormy Search for the Self by Stanislav Grof; Jeremy P. Tarcher, 1992

The Body Deva by Mary Mueller Shutan; Findhorn Press, 2018

The Hero with a Thousand Faces by Joseph Campbell; New World Library, 2008

The Seven Storey Mountain by Thomas Merton; Mariner Books, 1999

The Spiritual Awakening Guide by Mary Mueller Shutan; Findhorn Press, 2015

SECTION TWO

Living with Kundalini: The Autobiography of Gopi Krishna by Gopi Krishna; Shambhala, 1993

Play of Consciousness by Swami Muktananda; Siddha Yoga Publications, 2000

Raja Yoga by Swami Vivekananda; Vedanta Press, 1953

The Awakening of Intelligence by Jiddu Krishnamurti; Harper & Row, 1987

The Knee of Listening by Adi da Samraj; The Dawn Horse Press, 2004

The Varieties of Religious Experience by William James; online, 1902

SECTION THREE

Daughter of Fire by Irina Tweedie; The Golden Sufi Center, 1995

I Am That by Nisargadatta Maharaj; The Acorn Press, 2012

Mysticism by Evelyn Underhill; Dover Publications, 2002

Oasis of Stillness by Aghoreshwar Bhagwan Ramji; Aghor Publications, 1997

The Fourth Way by P.D. Ouspensky; Vintage, 1971

The Way of the Bodhisattva by Shantideva; Shambhala, 2006

Trials of the Visionary Mind by John Weir Perry; State University of New York press, 1998

SECTION FOUR

Center of the Cyclone by John Lilly; Ronin Publishing, 2007

Dark Night of the Soul by St. John of the Cross; Dover Publications, 2003

John Climacus: The Ladder of Divine Ascent by John Climacus; Paulist Pr, 1982

Talks with Ramana Maharshi: On Realizing Abiding Peace and Happiness by Ramana Maharshi; Inner Directions, 2000

Tao and Longevity by Huai-Chin Nan; Weiser Books, 1984

The Interior Castle by St. Teresa of Avila; Dover Publications, 2007

The Path of Purification by Bhadantacariya Buddhaghosa; Pariyatti Publishing, 2002

The Wings to Awakening by Thanissaro Bhikkhu; Dhamma Dana Publications, 2004

SECTION FIVE

Abdhidamma Studies: Buddhist Explorations of Consciousness and Time by Nyanaponika Thera; Wisdom Publications, 1998

Creative Meditation and Multi-Dimensional Consciousness by Lama Govinda; Theosophical Publishing House, 1976

Kundalini: Energy of the Depths by Lilian Silburn; State University of New York Press, 1988

Sat-Darshana Bhashya and Talks with Maharishi by Ramana Maharshi; Sri Ramanasramam, 2006

Spanda-Karikas: The Divine Creative Pulsation by Jaidevah Singh; Mozilla Banarsidass, 2014

Spiritual Life and the Word of God by Emanuel Swedenborg; Merchant Books, 2010

The Doctrine of Vibration by Mark Dyckowski; State University of New York Press, 1987

The Signature of All Things by Jacob Boehme; public domain

The Life Divine by Sri Aurobindo; Sri Aurobindo Ashram Press, 2006

Acknowledgments

Thank you to Mercury, Jeanne Gorham, Mary Murphy, and to Sara MB, all of whom have encouraged me to share what I know.

Thank you to my editor, Jane Ellen Combelic, for her clarity and insight.

Thank you to all of the clients, students, and colleagues who have helped shape this work.

About the Author

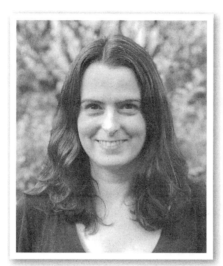

Photo by David H. Shutan

MARY MUELLER SHUTAN is a spiritual healer and teacher with an extensive background in various holistic health modalities including Chinese medicine, CranioSacral therapy, Zero Balancing, and shamanic healing. She is the author of *The Body Deva, Managing Psychic Abilities, The Complete Cord Course, The Shamanic Workbook I,* and *The Spiritual Awakening Guide*.

Mary lives near Chicago, Illinois. For more information on her work please visit her website: **www.maryshutan.com**

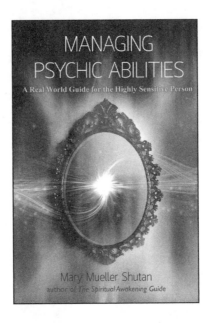

Managing Psychic Abilities
by Mary Mueller Shutan

APPROXIMATELY 20% OF THE POPULATION is sensitive or in some way psychic. Being sensitive or psychic can allow you to understand the world in a way that most people can't, and to see beyond what others are able to. But for many, sensitivities are a burden, causing overwhelm or even physical ailments. You don't want to become even more sensitive but know how to manage your life as it is.

This book can teach you how psychic abilities and sensitivities develop, where you are on the spectrum of these, and most importantly, the basic and intermediate skills and techniques you need to learn to be healthier, more functional, and to feel in control of your sensitivities and abilities.

The first modern guide on how to manage psychic abilities and sensitivities from a spiritual standpoint, this book will teach you everything you need to know so you can truly thrive in this world as a sensitive person.

978-1-84409-700-5

Also by this Author

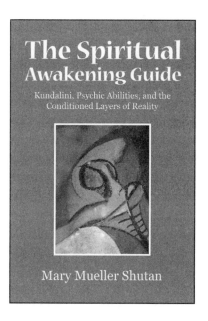

The Spiritual Awakening Guide
by Mary Mueller Shutan

THIS PRACTICAL BOOK opens new understandings of how to live in the world while going through an awakening process. Mary Mueller Shutan provides tools for how to navigate through each of the twelve layers of an awakened state and explains how to recognize where we are in our spiritual journey, along with common physical, emotional, and spiritual symptoms that may be experienced on the way. She offers the revolutionary idea that we are meant to be humans, to have a physical body with physical, sensate experiences and emotions. We are meant to live in the world and be a part of it even as fully awakened individuals.

This guide proposes a look at the possibility of leading a grounded, earthbound life of work, family, friends, and other experiences in an awakened state.

978-1-84409-671-8

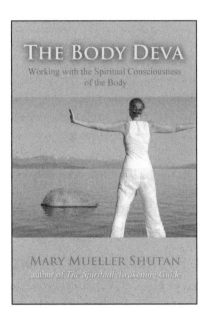

The Body Deva
by Mary Mueller Shutan

A STEP-BY-STEP GUIDE to understanding and working with the consciousness of your body, the body deva. Mary Mueller Shutan explains how our bodies hold the traumatic energies, emotions, physical issues, and restricting beliefs that cause us pain and feelings of disconnection. She details how to make contact and dialogue with our body deva to heal a variety of issues, from physical pains to ancestral and past life patterns to limiting ideas about what we can accomplish in this world.

By working with the body deva, she shows how we can discover the reasons why our pain, beliefs, or imbalances developed and resolve them to heal mind, body, and spirit, every layer of our being. She explores how to work with the archetypes, labels, limiting beliefs, and myths that underlie our unique history and reasons for being, and how to heal spiritual patterns through the physical body.

978-1-84409-745-6

F I N D H O R N   P R E S S

Life-Changing Books

Consult our catalogue online
(with secure order facility) on
www.findhornpress.com

For information on the Findhorn Foundation:
www.findhorn.org